in Psychiatry

Third Edition

Critical Reviews in Psychiatry
Third Edition

Edited by
Tom Brown &
Greg Wilkinson

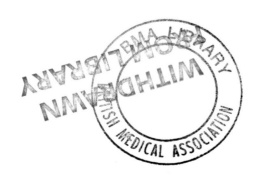

GASKELL

First edition ©1998 The Royal College of Psychiatrists
Second edition © 2000 The Royal College of Psychiatrists
© 2005 The Royal College of Psychiatrists
Reprinted 2007

British Library Cataloguing-in-Publication Data
A catalogue record for this book is available from the British Library.
ISBN 1-904671-15-2

Distributed in North America by Balogh International, Inc.

The views presented in this book do not necessarily reflect
those of the Royal College of Psychiatrists, and the publishers
are not responsible for any error or omission of fact. College
seminars are produced by the Publications Department of
the College; they should in no way be construed as providing
a syllabus or other material for any College Examination.

Gaskell is an imprint of the Royal College of Psychiatrists,
17 Belgrave Square, London SW1X 8PG.

The Royal College of Psychiatrists is a registered charity (no. 228636).

Typeset by Dobbie Typesetting Limited, Tavistock, Devon
Printed in Great Britain by Bell & Bain Limited, Thornliebank, Glasgow

Contents

Past papers and model answers

Contributors

Dr Tom Brown, Consultant Psychiatrist, Western Infirmary, Glasgow G11 6NT, UK

Dr Anne Cahill, Leeds Addiction Unit, 19 Springfield Mount, Leeds LS2 9NG, UK

Dr Anne-Marie Feeley, Glenmalure Day Hospital, Miltown Road, Dublin 6, Ireland

Dr Mona Freeman, Tavistock Clinic, 120 Belsize Lane, London NW3 5BA, UK

Professor Matthew Hotopf, Institute of Psychiatry, De Crespigny Park, Denmark Hill, London SE5 8AF, UK

Dr Rowena Jones, Queen Elizabeth Psychiatric Hospital, Edgbaston, Birmingham B15 2QZ, UK

Dr Helen Kenny, Little Woodhouse Hall, 18 Clarendon Road, Leeds LS2 9NT, UK

Ayla Khan, Early Psychosis Prevention & Intervention Centre (EPPIC), 35 Poplar Road, Parkville, Victoria 3052, Australia

Dr Stephen M. Lawrie, Senior Clinical Research Fellow, Department of Psychiatry, Royal Edinburgh Hospital, Edinburgh EH10 5FT, UK

Dr Andrew McIntosh, Lecturer in Psychiatry, Kennedy Tower, Royal Edinburgh Hospital, Morningside Park, Edinburgh EH10 5HF, UK

Dr Clementine Maddock, Maudsley Hospital, Denmark Hill, London SE5 8AZ, UK

Dr Philip Shaw, Maudsley Hospital, Denmark Hill, London SE5 8AZ, UK

Dr Danny H. Sullivan, Victorian Institute of Forensic Mental Health, Locked Bag 10, Fairfield, Victoria 3078, Australia

Paul Tiffin, Fleming Nuffield Unit, Burdon Terrace, Newcastle upon Tyne NE2 3AE, UK

Professor Greg Wilkinson, Department of Psychiatry, University of Liverpool, Liverpool L69 3GA, UK

Introduction

This book is aimed at psychiatrists in training who are taking the MRCPsych Part II Examination. We are pleased to include the first 11 MRCPsych Critical Review Papers in this third edition, along with model answers provided by prize-winning exam candidates.

Critical Review Paper

Psychiatrists should be able to evaluate published literature both in terms of its scientific validity and its clinical relevance. Good clinical practice is based on a combination of clinical judgement and sound application of research-based evidence, so pscyhiatrists need to acquire skills and confidence in critical appraisal of research and its application to their clinical work.

The Aims of the Critical Review Paper include:

(a) understanding research design and methodology;
(b) understanding sources of problems and bias in different kinds of research methodology;
(c) understanding basic statistics;
(d) definitions and meanings of measures important in critical appraisal, for example: sensitivity, specificity, odds ratio;
(e) knowledge of methodology of systematic reviews and meta-analysis;
(f) how to determine reliability and validity of results;
(g) (clinical relevance of) results in scientific papers;
(h) how to detect errors in research methodology and design;
(i) understanding the process and results of critical appraisal of a scientific paper;
(j) ability to suggest further experiments which would confirm or increase understanding in the field under investigation;
(k) placing important results of scientific papers in their clinical context and seeing how they might alter clinical practice.

Critical Reviews in Psychiatry

At the time we decided to produce the first edition of this book, as far as we were aware, there was no other book on the psychiatric aspects of critical review. We therefore wanted to produce a book which would be useful reading for all psychiatric trainees taking the MRCPsych Examination. We ourselves only had access to information from the College which was in the public domain and had seen no more than the two pilot papers produced by the College. As it turns out, the first and second editions proved highly successful.

Over time, the examination has matured and taken shape and we believe there is now sufficient material to provide a natural successor to the previous editions based directly on the examinations.

We are all very grateful to the authors of the specimen answers for their bravery in accepting our invitation to display their knowledge. We also thank the Examinations Department of the Royal College of Psychiatrists and the authors of the original papers on which the examinations were based for supporting our use of their work for this purpose. The Chief Examiner and colleagues on the Examinations Sub-Committee involved in the preparation of the MRCPsych Part II Examination played no other part in the preparation or production of this book.

Please note that our policy for this edition has been to present only the number of answers to a question requested by the examiners, even if there are other correct answers. This reflects current examination practice; for example, if a question asks for five examples, the examiner will ignore any answers given after the first five.

How to use this book

Begin by reading Lawrie's introductory chapter on EBM. In addition, we would particularly recommend the book by Sackett *et al* (1999) as a concise introductory text on evidence-based medicine. We also draw attention to Dr McIntosh's 'Trainee's Viewpoint' (pp. 9–10).

Critical Reviews in Psychiatry is structured as follows. Following the introductory material, there are 11 MRCPsych Critical Review Papers, each with model answers. We invite you to attempt each paper under 'exam conditions'.

Some tips

To make your task easier when you attempt these critical reviews – and the real thing – remember these tips.

(a) Read the question paper before reading the article for critical review.
(b) Prepare your thoughts using rough notes before answering the question paper and make sure you understand, in particular, the type of study and the subject of the investigation.
(c) Re-read each question carefully and make sure you tackle each component of it.
(d) Choose an order in which you wish to answer the questions posed, beginning with questions you can answer fully and at once and leaving until later those that may require more consideration.
(e) Look at the number of marks allotted to each question and allocate your time for each answer in the same proportion. For example, a question with 10 marks may have five components each with two marks or *vice versa*.
(f) Answer only the question that is being asked.
(g) Pay attention to the wording of the questions and structure your answers appropriately.
(h) Attempt an answer for each question.
(i) Write clearly and make your answer for each component of a question clear (using the appropriate numbers or headings) so that the examiner can properly evaluate your answer.
(j) Refer to established work (author, date) if you are confident it is relevant to your answer.

We hope you find *Critical Reviews in Psychiatry* interesting, useful and enjoyable. We would welcome receipt of all constructive criticism and comments directed at making improvements to future editions.

Tom M. Brown
Greg Wilkinson

Reference

Sackett, D., Straus, S. E., Richardson, W. S., *et al* (eds) (1999) *Evidence-Based Medicine: How to Practice and Teach EBM* (2nd edn). London: Churchill Livingstone.

Making sense of the numbers in evidence-based medicine
Stephen M. Lawrie

As doctors, we diagnose, treat and make prognoses about our patients. These decisions are guided by our training and clinical experience, but must be informed by important new research findings. Relevant studies must first be located, which is probably most effectively done by reading secondary publication sources such as the journal *Evidence-Based Mental Health*. Identified studies must then be 'critically appraised' in terms of scientific merit and clinical importance. Statistically significant results, even from rigorously conducted clinical research, are not necessarily clinically significant. For example, large treatment trials may report statistical differences, which might only benefit a small number of patients in clinical practice. The development of reliable and useful indices of clinical importance has been a central concern of the pioneers of the evidence-based medicine movement (Sackett *et al*, 1996, 1999). This brief review aims to explain these indices to a psychiatric audience.

Let's imagine that you have been asked by local general practitioners to provide useful information about the diagnosis, treatment and prognosis of depression in primary care. In particular, they want to know about a potential simple screening test, the efficacy of new antidepressants and how many patients will recover within one year. It just so happens that you are able to locate three relevant articles that look promising, and you set about devising clinically useful summary information.

Diagnosis

The hypothetical diagnosis paper evaluated the performance of a number of questions in identifying depressive illness as compared with the 'gold standard', that is, a structured psychiatric interview and diagnostic criteria. Crucially, all eligible subjects received both assessments from interviewers who were blind to the results of the other test. Let's say that many of the screening questions performed adequately, but the best balance of sensitivity and specificity was obtained with the simple question "Have you felt depressed for the past two weeks?" The performance of the screening and standard tests are shown in Table 1.

The screening question found 25 of the 30 patients identified as being depressed by the gold standard, and 60 of the 70 patients identified by the gold standard as not being depressed. These comparative

Table 1. Diagnosis. Gold standard diagnostic interview

	Depressed	Not depressed	Total
Screening question			
Depressed	25 (a)	10 (b)	35 (a+b)
Not depressed	5 (c)	60 (d)	65 (c+d)
Total	30 (a+c)	70 (b+d)	100 (N)

rates are the 'sensitivity' and 'specificity' of the screening question respectively, that is, the ability of the test to detect true positives and true negatives as judged by the gold standard. These can be expressed algebraically.

Equation 1

Sensitivity=a/(a+c), which in this example is 25/30=0.83, that is, 83% of people with the disease will test positive on the screening test.

Equation 2

Specificity=d/(b+d), which in this example is 60/70=0.86, that is, 86% of people without the disease will test negative on the test.

Sensitivity and specificity are properties of the test, whereas clinicians are interested in patients' results – of those patients who score as cases, how many actually have the disease and of those patients who score as non-cases, how many do not actually have the disease. These are the positive predictive values (PPVs) and negative predictive values (NPVs) respectively, which quantify the predictive power of particular test results.

Equation 3

PPV=a/(a+b), which in this example is 25/35=0.71, that is, 71% of those scoring positive on the test will actually have the disease.

Equation 4

NPV=d/(c+d), which in this example is 60/65=0.92, that is, 92% of those scoring negative on the test will actually not have the disease.

Unfortunately, the PPV and NPV are dependent on the prevalence of the disease. For example, if the prevalence of depression was only 10%, with similar sensitivity and specificity (as they are usually constant), the cell values in Table 1 would change (to approximately a=8, b=15, c=2 and d=75), the PPV would drop substantially (to about 8/23) and the NPV would increase (to about 75/77). Conversely, if the prevalence was higher, the PPV would increase and the NPV would fall. Few tests work well if the prevalence is less than 10% or more than 90%.

A useful way of summarising the performance of a diagnostic test regardless of prevalence is to calculate a likelihood ratio, as this can be done from the sensitivity and specificity. The likelihood ratio of a positive test result (LR+) is the likelihood that a positive test result comes from a person with the disease rather than one without; while the likelihood ratio of a negative result (LR−) is the likelihood that a negative test result comes from a person with the disease rather than one without.

Note that we are dealing with the 'odds' or relative probabilities of results in one group compared with another. It may help you to know that the probability of an event includes the observation in the numerator and denominator of the equation, whereas the odds of two events are represented separately in the numerator and denominator. For example, the probability of throwing any number with a die is one in six whereas the odds are one to five. Probabilities (P) and odds (O) are clearly related, such that P=O/(1+O) and O=P/(1−P).

Equation 5

LR+=[a/(a+c)]/[d/(b+d)], or sensitivity/(1−specificity), which in this example is 0.83/1−0.86=5.93, that is, a positive result is 5.93 times more likely to be found in a patient with the disease rather than one without.

Equation 6

LR−=[c/(a+c)]/[d/(b+d)], or (1−sensitivity)/specificity, which in this example is 1−0.83/0.86=0.20, that is, a negative result is 0.2 times more likely − or five times less likely − to be found in a patient with the disease than without.

The likelihood ratio, as a relative measure, is multiplied by the pre-test odds of having the disorder to generate the post-test odds. Probabilities are easier to interpret than odds, so the post-test odds are converted back into a post-test probability, that is, the probability that a person scoring positive (or negative) on the test actually has the disorder.

Equation 7

Pre-test odds=pre-test probability/(1−pre-test probability), which in this example is 0.3/(1−0.3)=0.43, that is, any patient is about a half as likely to have the disease as not. (It is worth noting that the pre-test probability is the same as the prevalence rate and that the pre-test odds are simply the rates in those with, relative to those without, the disease − 0.3 to 0.7.)

Equation 8

Post-test odds (of a positive result)=pre-test odds6LR+, which in this example is 0.4365.93=2.55, that is, a patient scoring positive on the test is 2.55 times more likely to have the disease than not.

Equation 9

Post-test probability (of a positive result)=post-test odds/(1+post-test odds), which in this example is 2.55/(1+2.55)=0.72, that is, 72% of patients scoring positive on the test will actually have the disease.

The same, rather laborious, calculations can be conducted for a negative test − prevalence is 0.3, pre-test odds 0.43, LR−0.20, post-test odds 0.086, post-test probability=0.079 (i.e. 7.9% of those scoring negative on the test will actually have the disease). Fortunately, nomograms are available to avoid the need for these calculations − as long as we know the LR+ and LR−, the pre-test probabilities are simply converted to post-test probabilities.

Returning to our hypothetical situation, you are now in a position to tell general practitioners that simply asking their patients if they have felt depressed for the past two weeks will mean that 72% of those responding positively will actually be depressed and that only 7.9% of those responding negatively will be falsely regarded as not depressed. Whether general practitioners regard this simple strategy as worthwhile might depend on their psychiatric experience, average consultation times and if there is a simple and safe therapeutic intervention for the identified cases.

Treatment

Any new treatment should ideally be evaluated in a randomised placebo-controlled double-blind trial, in which the outcomes of interest are measured in all subjects who enter the trial. Suppose that such a

Table 2. Treatment

	New antidepressant	Placebo	Total
Outcome			
Not depressed	40	20	60
Depressed	10	30	40
Total	50	50	100

trial compared the rates of treatment success, as measured by an arbitrary, but reliable 50% reduction in symptom levels, with a new antidepressant and a placebo in 100 patients with depression in a primary care setting. The hypothetical results are shown in Table 2.

Thus, 40 (80%) out of 50 patients treated with the new antidepressant responded as compared with 20 (40%) out of 50 patients treated with placebo. These are the experimental event rate (EER) and the control event rate (CER), respectively. The difference between them is likely to be statistically significant, but is it clinically important? The traditional measure of this is the proportional or relative risk reduction (RRR).

Equation 10

RRR=(EER−CER)/CER, which in this example is (80−40)/40=1 (or 100%), that is, antidepressants increase the relative response by 100%. (Note that, strictly speaking, this is a relative benefit increase (RBI) as a desirable event is being considered.)

The problem with the RRR (or RBI) is that it cannot distinguish large treatment effects from trivial effects. The RRR in this example would still be 1 if the EER and CER were 100% and 50% respectively and even if they were 2% and 1%. This is because the RRR does not consider the underlying chances of events (such as spontaneous recovery) in patients entering trials. In contrast, the simple difference between experimental and control event rates − the absolute risk reduction (ARR) − does allow for baseline risks.

Equation 11

ARR=EER−CER, which in this example is 80−40=40%, that is, antidepressants increase the absolute response rate by 40%. (Note that, strictly speaking, this is an absolute benefit increase (ABI) as a desirable event is being considered.)

Some readers will almost intuitively realise that if the average benefit is 40% then 2.5 (100/40) people will need to be treated to obtain recovery in one. This is the number needed to treat (NNT) and is simply calculated as the reciprocal of the ARR (or ARI).

Equation 12

NNT=1/ARR, which in this example is 1/0.4=2.5 (which is rounded up to 3.0 'whole' people).

This is the best estimate of the magnitude of the treatment effect from this hypothetical study, but when dealing with different patients from various populations we need to know the likely range of results. This is best expressed as a 95% confidence interval (95% CI), that is, the range of results within which we can be 95% confident or sure that the true value lies. There are a number of ways of calculating (usually approximate) confidence intervals, which also depend on the measure of interest, and one could not be expected to memorise them all. Interested readers are referred to Sackett *et al* (1997) for some of the more commonly used methods. It is, however, worth knowing that the confidence intervals on the NNT are simply the reciprocals of the confidence intervals on the ARR.

Equation 13

The 95% CI of the NNT is 1/higher confidence interval of the ARR to 1/lower confidence interval of the RR, which in this example is (using arbitrary values) 1/0.5 to 1/0.3=2 to 3.3 (rounded up to 4.0).

Provided an NNT is reasonably low, and the 95% CI around it is not too wide, one can be confident that a given intervention will work, in similar patients, in routine clinical practice. Whether a particular treatment was used will, however, also depend on likely adverse effects (and cost). Adverse effects can also be quantified, as a number needed to harm (NNH), in an analogous way to the NNT, that is, the NNH equals the reciprocal of the absolute difference in the rates of adverse events in the experimental and control groups.

Finally, as clinicians, we deal with individual patients rather than populations. Some of our patients are similar to those in randomised controlled trials but many are not. The NNT can be adapted for individual patients in a number of ways – with reference to our clinical experience, to the results of clinical audit or from figures in a prognosis paper on similar patients. The former technique is the easiest as it simply requires one to make an estimate of a patient's likely susceptibility to an outcome as compared to the average control patients in the reported trial. This estimate should be expressed as a decimal fraction (F) and divided into the NNT to produce an 'adjusted NNT'.

Equation 14

Adjusted NNT=NNT/F, which in this example if (say) a patient was judged to be half as likely to respond to antidepressants is 2.5/0.5=5.

The other techniques are likely to be more accurate, but are more difficult and time-consuming and are best used when considering whether a treatment reduces the rates of an undesirable event rather than increases the chance of a desirable one (see Sackett *et al*, 1996, 1999).

Returning to our general practitioners, you could inform them that they would need to treat three typical patients (confidence interval two to four patients) with the antidepressant to get one recovery that would have not occurred without treatment over the time scale of the trial.

Prognosis

Reliable data on prognosis is best obtained from (a meta-analysis of) cohort studies, where a group of patients at similar stages of their illness are prospectively followed-up for an adequate length of time to monitor the rates of outcomes of interest – such as recovery, relapse and death.

Suppose that such a study reported recovery rates from depression, in primary care, of 80% at one year. This is also the probability or chances of recovery. Note, however, that the confidence intervals around this estimate would need to be relatively narrow (say 70–90%) for this information to be clinically useful. Confidence intervals are actually quite simply calculated on probabilities (P) or proportions, such that it is worth running through the calculation of a 95% CI for this example.

Equation 15

The 95% CI of a proportion=$P \pm (1.96 \times$ the standard error). The standard error of a proportion is the square root of $[P \times (1-P)/N]$. In this example, the 95% CI is therefore $0.8 \pm (1.96 \times \sqrt{[0.8 \times (1-0.8)/100]}) = 0.8 \pm (1.96 \times \sqrt{[0.16/100]}) = 0.8 \pm (1.96 \times 0.04) = 0.8 \pm 0.08 = 0.72$ to 0.88 (or 72% to 88%).

Note that the standard error is heavily influenced by the size (n) of any study. If the same P was found in a study of 1000 subjects, the standard error would be about 0.01 and 95% CI would be approximately 70% to 82%. In other words, the larger a study is, the more confident one can be that the result is accurate.

Conclusions

At first glance, some of these concepts and calculations may seem a bit complicated. Relatively little practice, preferably in real-life clinical situations, will however, quickly accustom you to their use. In time, you will probably find them very useful, even essential, in guiding clinical decisions and communicating with your colleagues and your patients. They will certainly help you pass the membership exam and should facilitate your continuing professional development.

Acknowledgements

I thank Andrew McIntosh and Sanjay Rao for reading through a draft of this review.

References

Sackett, D. L., Richardson, S., Rosenberg, W., et al (eds) (1996) Evidence-Based Medicine: How to Practice and Teach EBM. London: Churchill Livingstone.

Sackett, D. L., Straus, S. E., Richardson, W. S., et al (eds) (1999) Evidence-Based Medicine: How to Practice and Teach EBM (2nd edn). London: Churchill Livingstone.

Further reading

Lawrie, S. M. & Geddes, J. R. (1998) Evidence-based medicine and psychiatry. In Edinburgh Companion to Psychiatric Studies (eds E. C. Johnstone, C. P. Freeman & A. Zealley). Pp. 865–877. Churchill Livingstone: Edinburgh.

Streiner, D. & Geddes, J. (1998) Some useful concepts and terms in articles about diagnosis. Evidence-Based Mental Health, 1, 6–7 (erratum in press).

Szatmari, P. (1998) Some useful concepts and terms used in articles about treatment. Evidence-Based Mental Health, 1, 39–40.

How to approach the MRCPsych Critical Review Paper. A trainee's viewpoint
Andrew McIntosh

What follows is based on my experience of sitting (and passing) the first Critical Review Paper. I found the experience enjoyable, useful and I've continued to use the methods since. The new paper tests the skills of the clinician in appraising published literature and then applying the evidence to their own practice. If you are sitting the exam you should be confident that it is not just a paper exercise, but a useful addition to your clinical skills that will help you decide whether the books and papers you read are valid, important and whether they can be used in caring for your patients. You should not be worried if you actually enjoy the experience!

The Critical Review Paper covers the use of articles on diagnosis, treatment, meta-analysis and systematic reviews, prognosis, economics, audit and clinical practice guidelines. Although the subject matter is familiar, some of the terms (such as NNT, likelihood ratios, confidence intervals) may seem daunting. Therefore, each area will need to be read and re-read many times before the concepts are finally grasped. Many people will read one or two of the books in the area (Brown & Wilkinson, 1998; Lawrie et al, 2000), although arguably this is one of the hardest ways of establishing confidence in the subject matter if it is done without any of the other methods mentioned below.

The most effective means of passing the exam is to begin to practise evidence-based medicine in your everyday work and to see the benefits and questions this raises about your own clinical practice. The following five-step plan is perhaps the ideal way to maximise your chances.

(a) Read one of the many texts. Don't worry about any of the mathematical terms you don't understand initially, these will become intuitive eventually with repeated practice. You will find that there is a great deal that you already understand or that is common sense.

(b) Join an evidence-based journal club. Ask yourself questions about the evidence for the interventions you make in your working day. Then find and appraise the evidence at the journal club. Using the journal club to learn from other people's clinical problems and appraisal of the literature will make this an efficient use of your time.

(c) Subscribe to, or read, the journal *Evidence-Based Mental Health* or other secondary publications such as *Clinical Evidence*. The journals publish critically appraised papers regularly, selecting only the most methodologically sound material. *Evidence-Based Mental Health* also includes a glossary and two brief pieces of an aspect of evidence-based psychiatry.

(d) Visit the many websites on evidence-based mental health (www.cebmh.com) or evidence-based medicine (www.cebm.net). The websites are useful reference guides and also include critically appraised topics (CATS) that are similar to the critical appraisal of published material that takes place at an evidence-based journal club.

(e) At least three months before the examination, start trying the sample questions included in this book. Save some questions to complete under exam conditions with others in your postgraduate class or study group. Get others to set questions under exam conditions: hopefully there will be teachers at your centre who will do this for you.

Finally, perhaps the most helpful means of passing the exam is to approach it with the right attitude. Those who see the 'evidence-based' approach as helpful and relevant will be more likely to enjoy the subject, pass the exam and continue using the methods in their own clinical practice afterwards. Your patients will also benefit from your efforts, therefore any time spent studying will not be wasted.

References

Brown, T. & Wilkinson, G. (2000) *Critical Reviews in Psychiatry* (2nd edn). London: Gaskell.

Lawrie, S. M., McIntosh, A. M. & Rao, S. (2000) *Critical Appraisal for Psychiatry.* Edinburgh: Churchill Livingstone.

PAST PAPERS AND MODEL ANSWERS

About the papers

The papers that follow are almost identical in content to those sat by candidates between spring 1999 and spring 2004. The exception to this is the Spring 1999 paper, to which a marking scheme has been added. The model answers have been written by the Laughlin prize-winning candidate/s for each paper. These papers are also available for a small fee from the Examinations Department at the Royal College of Psychiatrists, in a booklet that contains a commentary on each question, written by the examiners.

Guidance to candidates

Candidates are allowed **one and a half hours** to answer the whole paper. The paper has TWO questions and candidates are required to answer all parts of both questions. A total of 100 marks is allocated to the paper. There are 70 marks available for Question A and 30 marks for Question B. Each part of each question is worth 10 marks.

Candidates are advised to bring a calculator to the examination hall for this paper. Candidates are permitted to use a noiseless, cordless, pocket-sized non-programmable calculator without printout or graphic/word display facilities.

The Critical Review Paper is intended to assess skills and expertise which are not assessed in other parts of the MRCPsych Part II Examination. In the first part of the Examination (Question A) candidates will be asked to read a published paper, which will be presented in a condensed form, and will be required to answer questions about the findings of the paper, the design and methodology and the importance of the paper in affecting clinical practice. Question B is concerned with a shorter related research study, usually related to the first paper under discussion, and questions on this paper, many of which will be concerned with the practice of Evidence-Based Medicine, will be asked. Candidates will need to be aware of the science of research methodology and be skilled in the application of this. The knowledge and skills required include the following:

Knowledge

- Understanding of the most appropriate design and methodology to examine the hypothesis proposed in a research investigation.
- Recognition of the key features, and common sources of problems or bias, of different types of research methodology, including randomised controlled trials, cohort studies, case-control studies, single case studies, studies involving economic analysis and qualitative studies.
- Understanding of basic statistical concepts (confidence intervals and probability) with sufficient knowledge to be able to interpret the results from common statistical tests used for parametric data (e.g. t-tests, ANOVA, multiple regression) and non-parametric data (e.g. chi-squared test, Mann–Whitney U-test).
- Understanding of the definition and meaning of measures important in critical appraisal (including relative and absolute risk reduction, sensitivity, specificity, likelihood ratio, odds ratio and number needed-to-treat).
- Knowledge of the methodology of systematic reviews, including meta-analysis and the potential sources of bias in the interpretation of such analyses and overviews.

Skills

- The ability to determine the reliability and validity of information and results presented in a scientific paper.
- The ability to determine the clinical importance and relevance of results from the information given in a paper.

- The ability to detect errors in design and methodology that render the stated conclusions invalid or affect their impact.
- The ability to understand and assess logically the process and results of critical appraisal of such a paper.
- The capacity to suggest further experiments which would confirm or expand understanding in the field under investigation.
- The ability to place the results of the paper in clinical context and assess how far clinical practice may be altered as a consequence.

MRCPsych Part II Examination
Critical Review Paper
Spring 1999

Please read the instructions carefully before going further.

Instructions

1. This examination lasts for 90 minutes.
2. The paper has TWO questions Question A and Question B. You must attempt ALL parts of BOTH questions.
3. A total of 100 marks has been allocated to the whole paper. Each part of each question is worth 10 marks. Therefore, Question A is worth 70 marks, and Question B is worth 30 marks.
4. In answering Question A, candidates may wish to glance briefly at the questions they are asked to answer (on pages 20–21 of the paper), before reading the details of the research (described on pages 16–19).
5. Candidates are advised to bring a calculator to the examination hall for this paper. Candidates are only permitted to take a noiseless, cordless, pocket-sized non-programmable calculator WITHOUT printout or graphic/word display facilities.

Question A
A brief primary care intervention for problem drinkers
Scenario

You are working in a general psychiatry service within an inner city catchment area, characterised by a multi-cultural and fairly mobile population, and higher than average levels of unemployment. Talking with Dr Patel, one of the local general practitioners who also works as a clinical assistant in the acute hospital's accident and emergency department, you learn that there appear to be a disproportionately high number of attendances in the accident and emergency department attributable to alcohol-related problems. Dr Patel queries whether it would be possible for general practitioners to detect some of these problems earlier and, if so, whether they could intervene to reduce the levels of problem drinking and thus reduce the number of accident and emergency department attendances. Dr Patel has done a literature search, and has found the following paper, which he offers you for your opinion:

Fleming, M. F., Barry, K. L., Manwell, L. B., *et al* (1997) Brief physician advice for problem alcohol drinkers: a randomized controlled trial in community-based primary care practices. *Journal of the American Medical Association*, **277**, 1039–1045.

Read through the summary of the methods and results below, and then answer the questions which follow.

The paper

This paper describes a brief intervention for problem drinkers by primary care physicians in one mid-western state of the USA. The main aim was to determine whether a brief intervention by primary care physicians was better than an information booklet in reducing problem alcohol use among people attending their general practitioner.

Methodology
Background

The physicians who participated (*n*=64) had an average of 13 years of practice after qualification, and worked in a variety of primary care settings, from single-handed rural practices to large suburban clinics, but none in built-up urban areas. Over a two-year period, all their adult patients (aged 18–65 years) with scheduled appointments were asked by the practice receptionists to complete a screening questionnaire. Refusal rates varied considerably between clinics (mean 13%, range 2–30%). The questions were phrased in general terms to minimise the possible intervention effects of asking directly about alcohol use. Those patients who screened positive on the questionnaire were invited to participate in a 'Research Lifestyle Interview', conducted in the general practice clinic by one of 10 trained research interviewers. The interview was designed to gather information not only about alcohol use, its possible consequences and any previous treatment, but also about illicit drug use, past psychiatric history and family history. Patients who completed the interview procedures were each paid the equivalent of £30.

Eligibility criteria

Patients were eligible for the intervention if they consumed above threshold amounts of alcohol (13 drinks or 168 g alcohol per week for men, and 11 drinks or 132 g of alcohol per week for women). Exclusion criteria were:

(a) age below 18 or above 65 years;

(b) pregnancy;

(c) attendance at an alcohol treatment programme in the previous 12 months;

(d) reported symptoms of alcohol withdrawal in the previous 12 months;

(e) having received advice from their doctor about their drinking in the previous three months;

(f) consumption of more than 50 drinks per week;

(g) being judged suicidal on the basis of reported symptoms.

Patient sample

The age profile of those recruited reflected that of the community in which they lived. Eighty-eight per cent were Caucasian, 62% were married or cohabiting and 61% had received more than the compulsory level of education.

Patient allocation to the treatment groups

Patients who were eligible for inclusion in the study were randomised into either an experimental or a control group. Randomisation was carried out separately for men and women in each participating practice, using a computer-generated allocation method. Neither the doctors nor the practice staff knew which patients had been randomised to the control group.

Interventions

All patients who were recruited into the study received a booklet about general health matters. The patients in the control group received no other intervention for their drinking. Those randomised into the experimental group were invited to participate in two 15-minute interviews, one month apart with their own doctor, plus a follow-up telephone call from the practice nurse two weeks after the second interview. The intervention used a standard format, based on a workbook, and focused on general health as well as drinking alcohol and its effects. The doctors who took part in the study were all trained to use the intervention prior to the start of the research, and received at least two further 'booster' training sessions during the study.

Outcome assessments

Patients recruited into the study were followed up by telephone interviews six and 12 months after the intervention. For these follow-up interviews, the interviewers were rotated so that they did not interview the same patients as they had screened initially. The interviews focused on changes in alcohol use, health care utilisation and changes in health status. Family members were also contacted at 12 months to corroborate the patients' accounts. After the interviews, the patients' medical records were reviewed.

Results

Recruitment and follow-up

The patient flows are shown in Figure 1.

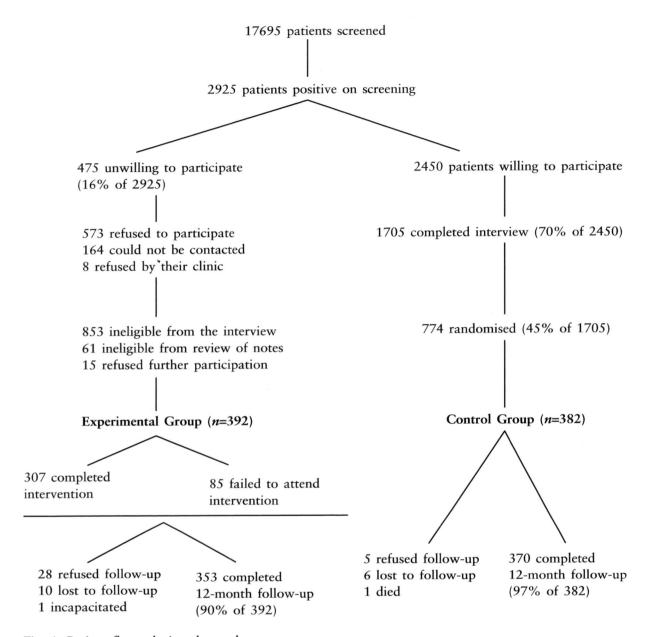

Fig. 1. Patient flows during the study

Identification by general practitioners of problem drinkers

At 12-month follow-up, only 50 control patients (13% of the group) reported that they had received an intervention for problem drinking from their general practitioner.

Alcohol consumption

Table I shows the number of episodes of binge drinking in the 30 days prior to each assessment (binge drinking was defined as >4 drinks for women and >5 drinks for men on a single occasion). Note that information in all the tables is given in the same format as in the published paper.

Table 1. Participants who were binge drinking in the 30 days prior to each assessment

	Treatment (n=392)		Control (n=382)			
	n	%	n	%	t	P
Baseline	288	85	317	87	0.44	NS
6 months	200	59	266	73	3.77	<0.001
12 months	188	56	261	71	4.33	<0.001

Table 2 shows the number of episodes of excessive drinking in the seven days prior to each assessment (excessive drinking was defined as >20 drinks per week for men and >13 drinks per week for women).

Table 2. Participants who drank excessively in the seven days prior to each assessment

	Treatment (n=392)		Control (n=382)			
	n	%	n	%	χ^2	P
Baseline	160	47	176	48	0.26	NS
Six months	67	20	115	31	3.52	<0.001
12 months	60	18	119	33	4.53	<0.001

Accident and emergency department attendance

Self-reported accident and emergency department attendance is shown in Table 3.

Table 3. Number of participants who reported attending the accident and emergency department in the six months prior to each assessment

	Treatment (n=392)		Control (n=382)			
	n	%	n	%	χ^2	P
Self-reported No. of emergency department visits (No. of patients) in last 6 months						
Baseline	75	58	80	65	2.45	>0.10
6 months	47	40	70	56		
12 months	60	47	62	50		

Question A

NOTE: Each question is worth 10 marks. There are a total of 100 marks for the whole paper, 70 marks for Question A and 30 marks for Question B.

Question A1

List five features of the design of this study which contribute to the strengths of its methodology.

[2 marks for each feature up to a maximum of 10 marks]

Question A2

For each feature listed above, explain briefly how it contributes to the strengths of the study design.

[2 marks for each feature up to a maximum of 10 marks]

Question A3

List *four* potential or actual weaknesses of the study design.

[3 marks, 3 marks, 2 marks, 2 marks]

Question A4

Summarise as precisely and as accurately as you can the main results as they have been given in the tables.

[10 marks]

Question A5

Considering only excessive drinking at 12 months (Table A2): what is the relative rate reduction (RRR) due to the intervention? (As well as giving the RRR, show how you calculate this.)

[10 marks]

Question A6

Considering only excessive drinking at 12 months (Table A2):

(a) What is the absolute rate reduction (ARR) and how do you calculate this?

[5 marks]

(b) If you were a Wisconsin general practitioner introducing this intervention, to how many people would you need to offer it to have one patient with a successful outcome?

[5 marks]

Question A7

Dr Patel's original query was whether local general practitioners might be able to detect alcohol-related problems earlier and intervene to reduce alcohol-related accident and emergency visits. What would you say to him about the applicability of this paper to his query?

[10 marks]

Question B

The following table is taken from a study of 521 patients admitted to medical or orthopaedic wards of a single general hospital. The ability of the CAGE questionnaire to predict alcohol-related problems (alcohol abuse or alcohol dependence, both operationally defined) was compared using a rigorous diagnostic interview as the 'gold standard'.

No. of positive CAGE responses	Alcohol abuse/dependence		Sensitivity	Specificity	Positive predictive value
	Present	Absent			
0	18	358	—	—	—
1	11	28	0.85	0.89	0.62
2	26	14	0.73	0.93	0.82
3	37	1	0.51	0.997	0.99
4	23	0	0.20	1.00	1.00
Total	117	401			

Question B1

The chairman of your local Community Health Council (a lay person with little medical knowledge) has been given a copy of this table during a discussion on alcohol problems. He wants to know what the results mean. How would you briefly summarise the table for him, and interpret its results?

[10 marks]

Question B2

To use the questionnaire, you need to define how many positive responses the patient needs to give before being classified as having alcohol-related problems in screening. If you were applying the CAGE questionnaire as a screening tool in clinical practice in a general hospital setting, what cut-off point would you select?

[10 marks]

Question B3

What would be the consequences of choosing this cut-off point, in terms of people without alcohol-related problems screening positive on the CAGE, and people with alcohol-related problems being missed?

[10 marks]

Model answers by Rowena Jones

Question A1

1. Concealed allocation.
2. Randomised.
3. Controlled.
4. Prospective.
5. Intervention standardised.

Question A2

1. Concealed allocation – in this paper the randomisation was generated by a computer. This ensures that the randomisation schedule is not known to the investigators and therefore they cannot influence who will be allocated to which group.

2. Randomised – this ensures that allocation to the treatment or control groups is by chance alone, and that the two groups should therefore be similar in all other respects apart from the intervention. Men and women were randomised separately to ensure an equal number in each group. This would remove the problem of sex being a confounding factor in the results.

3. Controlled – the control group is present to be used as a comparison, so that any change in outcome for the experimental group can be directly attributable to the intervention. Controlled trials use hypotheticodeductive reasoning to attempt to falsify, rather than confirm, the null hypotheses.

4. Prospective – prospective studies are much less susceptible to bias than retrospective ones, as recall bias is eliminated. Prospective randomised controlled trials are the design of choice for studies about therapy.

5. Standardisation of the intervention minimises biases due to variation in the intervention being delivered. The GPs received structured and repeated training and the intervention was manualised.

Question A3

1. Recruitment bias – the study only picks up those with scheduled appointments, and out of those who were eligible on initial screening there was a high refusal rate.

2. Generalisability – the study is conducted at rural and suburban GP practices and therefore the findings may not be applicable to multi-cultural urban practices.

3. The study is not placebo-controlled. The control group only received a booklet – it would have been preferable for them to have received a time-matched health intervention from the GPs. This discrepancy means that a change in the treatment group compared with the control could be attributed to non-specific factors such as extra time spent with the GP.

4. The study is not blind. The patients and doctors were not blinded, although it does state that the doctors did not know which patients were in the control group. Although the interviewers were rotated so that they did not re-interview the same patients it does not state that they were blinded as to the research status of the patients. Lack of blinding may result in ascertainment bias.

Question A4

Results appear to have been analysed on an intention-to-treat basis.

Table 1 – The two groups were similar at the start of the study period. The rate of binge drinking over the preceding 30 days in the treatment group was significantly reduced at 6 months follow-up compared with the control group. This difference was maintained at 12-month follow-up.

Table 2 – The rate of excessive drinking over the preceding 7 days was significantly reduced at 6-month follow-up compared with the control group. Again this difference was maintained at 12-month follow-up.

Table 3 – There is no significant difference between the study and control groups in terms of numbers of A&E visits during the study period.

Question A5

RRR = the rate reduction in the treatment group divided by the rate reduction in the control group.
Rate reduction in the treatment group $= 0.47 - 0.18 = 0.29$
Rate reduction in the control group $= 0.48 - 0.33 = 0.15$
RRR $= 0.29/0.15 = 1.9$.

Question A6

(a) ARR is the rate reduction in the treatment group minus the rate reduction in the control group.
$0.29 - 0.15 = 0.14$.

(b) If you were a Wisconsin general practitioner introducing this intervention, to how many people would you need to offer it to have one patient with a successful outcome?
$NNT = 1/0.14 = 7$

Question A7

1. The paper does not address Dr Patel's specific query as to whether GPs might be able to detect alcohol problems earlier. GP detection of harmful drinking is low in this paper – only 13% of the control group reported that they had received an intervention for problem drinking at 12-month follow-up. This suggests that the intervention may not be given to those who would benefit from it.

2. The study may not be generalisable to GPs local to Dr Patel, who work in inner city multi-cultural areas.

3. The intervention in the paper delivered by GPs can reduce binge drinking and excessive drinking in drinkers but there is no evidence that it reduces A&E visits.

Question BI

The table gives information on the practicability of using the CAGE questionnaire to predict alcohol-related problems in medical and surgical hospital in-patients. Cut-off scores from 1 to 4 on the CAGE are compared in terms of their likelihood of picking up alcohol-related problems. The measures given are the sensitivity, specificity and positive predictive value. Sensitivity means the percentage of those who have alcohol problems that test positive on the CAGE, i.e. the true positives. Specificity means the percentage of those without alcohol problems who are correctly found negative. Positive predictive value means the percentage of those found positive on the test that do indeed have alcohol problems. Using a cut-off score of 1 positive response on the CAGE, the sensitivity and specificity are both reasonably high, at 0.85 and 0.89 respectively. The positive predictive value, however, is only 0.62, meaning that only 62% of those testing positive will actually have an alcohol problem.

As the cut-off score on the CAGE is raised, the sensitivity of the test falls. This means that more patients with alcohol problems will be missed. The specificity of the test rises. This means that fewer people will be wrongly identified as having an alcohol problem. At the same time, the positive predictive value of the test rises, meaning that the percentage of people scoring positive who actually have an alcohol problem increases.

Question B2

An ROC curve of sensitivity plotted against $1 - $ specificity can be used to determine the optimum cut-off point. However, this also depends on the purpose for which the questionnaire is being used. If it is being used as a screening tool then you are most interested in a test with high sensitivity, to ensure that individuals with alcohol problems are not missed. A cut-off score of 1 would provide this by maximising the sensitivity. Even though you will have a high false-positive rate, further tests with higher specificity can then be considered for those who screen positive.

Question B3

Choosing a cut-off point of 1 would mean that the number of people with alcohol-related problems that were missed would be minimised at the expense of falsely identifying more people without alcohol-related problems as cases.

From the data given, a cut-off of 1 would mean that 43 people would be falsely identified as having alcohol problems, while 18 with alcohol-related problems would be missed.

MRCPsych Part II Examination
Critical Review Paper
Autumn 1999

Please read the instructions carefully before going further.

Instructions

1. This examination lasts for 90 minutes.
2. The paper has TWO questions, Question A and Question B. You must attempt ALL parts of BOTH questions.
3. A total of 100 marks has been allocated to the whole paper. Each part of each question is worth 10 marks. Therefore, Question A is worth 70 marks, and Question B is worth 30 marks.
4. In answering Question A, candidates may wish to glance briefly at the questions they are asked to answer (on pages 30–31 of the paper), before reading the details of the research (described on pages 26–28).
5. Candidates are advised to bring a calculator to the examination hall for this paper. Candidates are only permitted to take a noiseless, cordless, pocket-sized non-programmable calculator WITHOUT printout or graphic/word display facilities.

Question A
Long-term prognosis in schizophrenia

Mr Alan James, an 18-year-old man, is admitted to hospital with a six-week history of third person auditory hallucinations, agitation and passivity feelings. He had previously been well, with no past history of psychiatric disturbance. He denies any drug abuse and a drug screen following admission proves negative. The working diagnosis is schizophrenia. Mr James's parents ask for an interview with you to discuss their son's prognosis. The first question they want to ask is: 'what is the overall outcome likely to be over the next 10 years?' A second question concerns the effects of negative symptoms on the outcome. Through a colleague at work, Mr James's father has made contact with another family who have a son with schizophrenia. Apparently, this young man has shown negative symptoms and has remained unwell for some years. When the parents come to see you, they bring with them a copy of a paper they have found via the internet. Read through the summary of the paper below, then answer the questions which follow.

Mason, P., Harrison, G., Glazebrook, C., *et al* (1995) Characteristics of outcome of schizophrenia at 13 years. *British Journal of Psychiatry*, **167**, 596–603.

Background

The patients studied in this paper were first identified in the International Pilot Study of Schizophrenia, which examined the determinants of outcome of schizophrenia in 15 countries. Nottingham, where the present study is based, was the UK centre for the International Pilot Study.

Sample
Original sample

During the two-year period 1 August 1978 to 31 July 1980, all patients between the ages of 15 and 54 years making their first-ever contact with psychiatric services in Nottingham (population 390 000) were screened. Screening included not only those who were admitted as in-patients, but also every other type of contact with services. All eligible patients were interviewed by a research psychiatrist, using (amongst other assessment instruments) the Present State Examination. After the assessments had been completed, at least two project psychiatrists together with the researchers who had conducted the interviews discussed all the available information on each patient to reach a consensus diagnosis, using ICD–9 criteria. This procedure identified 67 patients (22 women, 45 men) who could be assigned a project diagnosis of schizophrenia. The investigators also checked the Nottingham Psychiatric Case Register, general practitioners and private psychiatric hospitals near Nottingham to identify patients who should possibly have been included in the study but were not identified by the procedures used. Of nine such cases identified, only three were judged to fall into 'certain' or 'very likely' categories of schizophrenia.

Follow-up sample

Most patients in the original sample were traced using the Nottingham Psychiatric Case Register and the Medical Records Department at Mapperley Hospital, Nottingham. Others were found using the Electoral Register and the Registrar for Births, Deaths and Marriages. Use was also made of the National Health Service Central Register and various Family Health Services Authorities throughout the country. It was possible to trace 63 of patients in the original sample (94%). Of the patients traced, five (8%) had died, three following suicide and another under circumstances suggesting suicide. Of the remaining 58 patients, high quality information could be obtained either by face-to-face interview or through records and informants on 54 patients (94%).

Face-to-face interviews were conducted with 48 patients (83% of 58) and two further patients (3%) were interviewed by telephone. No significant differences were found between the 58 patients who completed follow-up, those lost to follow-up (N=4) and those who died (N=5) in age, sex, marital status, type of onset, or initial Present State Examination profile.

Assessments

The following instruments were used:

(a) Present State Examination (PSE): the CATEGO computer programme was used to determine the number of subjects who met the restrictive definition of schizophrenia (CATEGO Class S+), at entry and at follow-up.

(b) Scale for the Assessment of Negative Symptoms (SANS): The SANS was used to determine thenumber of patients who had negative symptoms during the month before the follow-up assessment. A SANS summary score of greater than 2 indicates the presence of negative symptoms.

(c) Life Chart Schedule (LCS): This codes symptoms, treatment, residency and employment history for the two years prior to the assessment, and for the entire follow-up period.

(d) Disability Assessment Schedule (DAS): The information used from this scale included the adjusted score for Dysfunctional Overall Behaviour (derived from scores for social withdrawal and self-care).

Information for each assessment was gathered from both the patient and a key informant, and further information was elicited from general practice records and hospital records.

Results

Symptoms

At entry to the study, 70% of the patients were classified according to the CATEGO programme as S+ (i.e. meeting a restrictive definition of schizophrenia). At follow-up, only 19% of those assessed were classified at S+. Of the patients assessed at follow-up with the SANS, 48% had summary scores greater than 2 (i.e. showed clinically important negative symptoms in the months prior to follow-up). Twenty-seven of those assessed at follow-up (47%) showed evidence of negative symptoms in the two years prior to the follow-up assessment.

Course of the illness

Table I summarises the course of the illness in the two years prior to the follow-up assessment, separately for the whole sample and for those patients (N=27) who had shown negative symptoms in the two years prior to the follow-up assessment.

Table 1. Course of illness and negative symptoms in the two years prior to the follow-up assessment (percentages in parentheses)

Type of course	Total sample	Negative symptoms in the 2 years prior to the follow-up assessment	
		Present	Absent
Episodic	6 (10)	3 (50)	3 (50)
Continuous	20 (34)	16 (80)	4 (20)
Neither episodic nor continuous	2 (3)	2 (100)	1 (0)
Never psychotic	30 (52)	6 (20)	24 (80)
Total	58	27 (47)	31 (53)

Disability

Information from the Disability Assessment Schedule was available on 55 subjects. Of these, 24 (44%) showed no dysfunction in overall behaviour and 23 (43%) showed no dysfunction in their social roles.

Complete recovery

If this is defined as meaning that the patient is alive at follow-up with no symptoms, no disability and on no treatment, then 11 (17%) of the sample available for follow-up had recovered completely at 13 years.

Associations between negative and other symptoms

Table 2 shows the association between negative symptoms at follow-up assessment, and: (a) overall psychotic symptoms at follow-up; (b) psychotic symptoms which had been continuous during the two years prior to the follow-up assessment.

Table 2. Association between negative symptoms and overall psychotic symptoms at follow-up

	Negative symptoms at follow-up assessment		Total	Odds ratio (95% CI)*	χ^2 (p)
	Present	Absent			
Overall psychotic symptoms at follow-up					
Present	17	8	25	6.0 (1.5–26.2)	6.9 (p<0.01)
Absent	6	17	23		
Total	23	25	48		
Continuous psychotic symptoms for 2 years prior to follow-up					
Present	16	5	21	9.1 (2.1–43.9)	10.0 (p<0.01)
Absent	7	20	27		
Total	23	25	48		

*95% CI, 95% confidence interval of odds ratio.

Question B

Mortality of a cohort of patients with schizophrenia

The following data are taken from Anderson *et al, British Journal of Psychiatry,* **159** (suppl. 13), 30–33, 1991.

All patients discharged from in-patient or day-patient care at Northwick Park Hospital near London in the 11-year period 1 January 1975 to 1 January 1985 were followed up between two to five years after discharge. The case notes were examined and those that fulfilled the St Louis criteria for schizophrenia formed the study sample. After this procedure 532 cases were identified, of which 291 were men and 241 were women.

At the time of enquiry on 1 January 1989, 382 of these patients were known to be alive, 69 were dead and 81 could not be traced. Of the 69 deaths, 40 died of natural causes whereas 24 deaths were unnatural. The five remaining deaths could not be clearly classed as natural or unnatural. However, only 7 of the 24 deaths were adjudged to be due to suicide with 15 recorded as an open verdict (no decision made about cause) in the Coroner's Court. Two patients had no inquest and no decision was made about the cause of death in these individuals.

The frequency of all causes of death, including suicide and myocardial infarction recorded separately, is shown in Table 1. The expected mortality of the general population living in the same district health authority during the period under enquiry was calculated separately. The subject-years method was used to calculate the expected number of deaths among the cohort with schizophrenia.

Table 1. Standardised mortality rates (SMR) for all causes of death, death due to myocardial infarction and death attributed to suicide

Cause of death	Women			Men		
	Deaths (N)	SMR	95% CI* of SMR	Deaths (N)	SMR	95% CI* of SMR
All causes of death	30	2.57	1.73–3.64	39	2.44	1.75–3.34
Death due to myocardial infarction	7	2.83	1.14–5.83	6	1.42	0.52–3.09
Suicide (whole sample)**	2	12.77	1.53–46.13	5	19.5	6.22–44.7
Suicide (patients aged 15–44 years)	2	29.25	3.51–105.6	4	27.85	7.5–71.3
Suicide (patients aged over 44 years)	0	—	—	1	8.51	0.21–47.4

*95% confidence interval.
**Using suicide verdicts only.

Question A

NOTE: Each question is worth 10 marks. There are a total of 100 marks for the whole paper, 70 marks for Question A and 30 marks for Question B.

Question AI

(i)   What type of study design is used in the study described in the paper?

[2 marks]

(ii)   What alternative study designs could be used to determine the prognosis of a first episode of schizophrenia?

[2 marks for each, up to a maximum of 4 marks]

(iii)   For each study design you mention, give one advantage and one disadvantage of its use.

[1 mark for each advantage, 1 mark for each disadvantage]

Question A2

(i)   List *two* strengths of the design of this study. Take care to distinguish between the study design and its execution; only the former is relevant here. Do not include any points you may have mentioned in answering Question AI.

[4 marks for each, up to a maximum of 8 marks]

(ii)   For each point you list, explain why it is a strength.

[1 mark for each explanation, up to a maximum of 2 marks]

Question A3

(i)   Only 54 of the 67 patients in the original cohort could be assessed at follow-up by 'high quality information'. How far does this affect the conclusions in the paper?

[4 marks]

(ii)   Explain your reasoning.

[2 marks for each explanation, up to a maximum of 6 marks]

Question A4

Summarise five points from the results from Table I which can contribute to answering the first question posed by Mr James's parents (what is the longer-term outcome likely to be)?

[2 marks for each answer, up to a maximum of 10 marks]

Question A5

(i)   What do the results of Table 2 show about the relationship between outcome and the presence or absence of negative symptoms? Please state *two* main findings.

[3 marks each, up to a maximum of 6 marks]

(ii)   What information in the table allows you to judge how certain you can be about these findings?

[4 marks]

Question A6

The results in Table I show that over 50% of the original cohort were not psychotic during the two-year period before follow-up assessment. Please give five possible reasons to explain these results.

[2 marks for each, up to a maximum of 10 marks]

Question A7

(i)   Assume that, instead of being admitted to a psychiatric unit, Mr James had been taken to see his general practitioner who had decided to treat Mr James himself with an antipsychotic drug, because Mr James and his family were very resistant to referral to psychiatric services. In this event, how far are the results of the present study applicable?

[2 marks]

(ii)   Give *four* reasons for your answer.

[2 marks each, up to a maximum of 8 marks]

Question B

Question BI

(i)   Define standardised mortality rate (or ratio) (SMR).

[6 marks]

(ii)   Using the data in Table I, how many deaths would have been expected among (a) *all* men and (b) *all* women, of the same age distribution as the study sample with schizophrenia, in the catchment area of the district health authority in which the patients resided?

[2 marks for each, up to a maximum of 4 marks]

Question B2

(i)   The mortality rate in women from myocardial infarction appears greater than in men. Is this difference statistically significant?

[2 marks]

(ii)   Explain the reasons for your choice.

[3 marks]

(iii)   Is the mortality rate in women from myocardial infarction significantly different statistically from that of the general population?

[2 marks]

(iv)   Explain your reasonsing.

[3 marks]

Question B3

(i)   Twenty-four deaths were considered unnatural. The majority was given open verdicts (no decision made about cause). In the light of this, comment on the use of suicide verdicts only in the calculation of SMR for patients with schizophrenia.

[4 marks]

(ii)   Summarise the results concerned with suicide verdicts shown in Table BI. Please list *three* main findings.

[2 marks for each, up to a maximum of 6 marks]

Model answers by Paul Tiffin

Question A1

(i)   This is a longitudinal or cohort study. As the subjects included were assembled at the same stage in the course of the illness (i.e. at first episode) prior to follow-up it is an inception cohort study.

(ii)   Case studies and case series are often the first sources of information on the natural history of a disorder, but these are not discussed here as they produce qualitative rather than quantitative data and are not 'study designs' as such. Cohort studies, being prospective in nature, are the investigation of choice when studying the course of a disorder. However, at least two less suitable designs could contribute useful data when broadly investigating the prognosis of a first episode of psychosis.
    1.   A case–control study; for example, this could match subjects who have demonstrated a poor outcome from a first episode of schizophrenia with those who have not. The characteristics of these two groups could then be compared to retrospectively evaluate factors which may be particularly associated with either a poor or a good prognosis.
    2.   An experimental study design such as a randomised controlled trial (RCT) could also be used, where differing interventions are used in different groups following a first episode of schizophrenia, in order to assess whether the prognosis is influenced in any way. For example, following the initial episode one group may receive standard case management and medication while another group could receive an additional family intervention aimed at reducing the level of expressed emotion (EE). Follow-up would evaluate the course and prognosis in both groups.

(iii)   Case–control study:
Advantages – It would be easier to ascertain the cases, with no need to wait for the follow-up time to elapse or trace the subjects.

Disadvantages – The diagnosis and details of the cases will be retrospective in nature and probably not standardised. This will introduce recall bias and diminish reliability when evaluating previous symptoms. Matching the two groups to try to avoid confounding factors could prove difficult in practice. In general, case–control studies are used for investigating the causation of a disorder and are particularly useful in this respect in relatively rare conditions where cohort studies are less practical.

Experimental study:
Advantages – In addition to evaluating the course and prognosis of the illness in the subjects, data would be collected which would be of practical value in selecting interventions that could potentially modify the long-term outcome.

Disadvantages – Matching such groups to eliminate potential confounding factors can be difficult. Also, it may be unethical to withhold from a control group interventions that are known or strongly suspected to be of benefit. In practice it is highly unlikely that such a design would be used for primarily determining the prognosis of a disorder.

Question A2

(i)   Strengths of the design include:
1.   The inclusion of a screening procedure in order to ascertain cases.
2.   The use of a prospective, rather than retrospective, diagnosis of schizophrenia.

(ii)
1.   The use of a screening procedure would make it more likely that patients in the study area presenting with a first-episode of psychosis would be detected and included in the study, leading to a more representative sample.
2.   The use of a prospective diagnosis would prevent the introduction of recall bias when making a diagnosis of schizophrenia.

Question A3

(i)   This is unlikely to affect the conclusions dramatically.

(ii)   Fifty-four of the 67 patients constitutes 80.5% and, overall, 94% of the original sample were traced. These are reasonably high rates given the 13-year period of follow-up and would be generally regarded as acceptable for this type of study. In addition to the 54 patients for whom 'high quality information' was obtained, four patients, although unavailable for interview, had information available from their notes and records and these may have provided adequate data to estimate their course and prognosis reasonably accurately. Taking this into account, data were available on 87% of the original cohort at follow-up and are thus relatively complete.

The paper states that those that were lost to follow-up did not differ from those who remained in the study with regard to their demographic characteristics and baseline Present State Examination profile. This means that it is less likely that those subjects not followed up comprised a specific sub-group of patients who differ dramatically from the remaining cohort and whose exclusion would significantly influence the final findings.

It could, however, still be hypothesised that those who were lost to follow-up could have differed in their prognosis, even if their characteristics at baseline assessment did not differ markedly from the remaining cohort. For example, those four patients who were thought to have died by suicide may have been affected by more severe symptoms than the group as a whole. Conversely, other patients lost to follow-up may have experienced less severe symptoms, leading to loss of contact with health services or even enabled emigration out of the UK. Nevertheless, as long as there is a mixture of different outcomes in those subjects lost to follow-up they are unlikely to significantly influence the overall conclusions. The fact that there were different reasons for the loss of subjects to follow-up makes such heterogeneity in those lost to the study more likely.

Question A4

Relevant points include:
1. 10% of the overall sample demonstrated an episodic course to their illness over the two years prior to the follow-up at 13 years.
2. Approximately a third of the subjects (34%) demonstrated a continuous course to their illness in the 2 years prior to the follow-up point.
3. 47% of patients demonstrated negative symptoms in the 2 years prior to the follow-up assessment.
4. Just over half the subjects (52%) were never psychotic in the 2-year period prior to follow-up.
5. 3% of patients followed a course of illness which was neither episodic or continuous in the 2 years prior to follow-up.

I have not commented on 'disability' or 'complete recovery' values, although they are relevant to the question posed by Mr James' parents, as these do not appear to be part of Table A1. Also, I have not focused on the association between poor outcome and negative symptoms apparent in the figures in the table, as this is more relevant in addressing the parent's second question rather than their first. The table does not contain any indication of the statistical significance of the values, and therefore this cannot be commented on.

Question A5

(i)   The results demonstrate a statistically significant association between the presence of overall psychotic symptoms at follow-up and the detection of negative symptoms at follow-up. For example, of the 25 subjects who demonstrated overall psychotic symptoms at follow-up, 17 (68%) were reported as also having negative symptoms. Conversely, of the 23 subjects who were free of overall psychotic symptoms at follow-up, 17 (74%) were reported as not having negative symptoms at this time.

The results also demonstrate a statistically significant association between the presence of continuous psychotic symptoms at 2 years prior to follow-up and the detection of negative symptoms at follow-up. For example, of the 21 subjects who demonstrated continuous psychotic symptoms at follow-up, 16 (76%) were reported as also having negative symptoms. Conversely, of the 27 subjects who did not have continuous psychotic symptoms prior to the follow-up period, 20 (74%) were reported as having absent negative symptoms.

These findings are consistent with a concept of the presence of negative symptoms representing a marker for a poorer prognosis in terms of the course of psychotic symptoms. According to this study, the presence of negative symptoms significantly increases the chances of a patient experiencing chronic or continuous psychotic symptomatology.

(ii)
1. The 95% confidence intervals for the odds ratio (OR); these display the limits within which we are 95% confident that the true OR lies (i.e. if the study were to be repeated 100 times we would expect the resulting ORs to fall within these limits at least 95 times). When the 95% confidence intervals do not overlap the value 1.0, they indicate a statistically significant difference in the outcome measure between the groups with and without the risk factor being investigated (i.e. we can be 95% certain that the difference in

outcomes did not occur as a result of chance). However, in the case of Table A2, although the 95% confidence intervals for the ORs do not overlap 1.0, they are relatively wide and therefore are less reassuring regarding the accuracy of the high ORs portrayed (6.0 and 9.1 respectively) than a narrow range would be, despite indicating the statistical significance of the findings.

2. The chi-squared value (χ^2) and corresponding p value; the chi-squared test takes the observed proportions of subjects in the relevant cells of the table and compares these with those that would be expected by chance if no differences existed between the experimental groups. The corresponding p value indicates the probability that the observations could have occurred by chance. A smaller p value therefore represents an increased probability that a true difference exists between the two groups. A p value of 0.05 or less is conventionally taken as the cut-off for accepting that an observed difference is significant (i.e. there is a one in twenty probability that the observation occurred by chance) but a smaller value must be used in order to increase the stringency or, for example, to correct for the effects of multiple testing.

Question A6

Possible reasons include (not necessarily in order of likelihood):

1. The initial diagnosis of schizophrenia was incorrect in some of the study subjects. The psychotic symptoms detected at baseline were thus not representative of a chronic mental illness and were not present at follow-up, after the initial episode had resolved.
2. The study failed to detect chronic psychotic symptoms where they were in fact present. For example, the subjects may have been able to conceal psychotic experiences from the investigators or otherwise failed to disclose them.
3. The subjects had received treatment which had ameliorated their psychotic symptoms by the time of the follow-up period or had spontaneously recovered without treatment.
4. The psychotic symptoms experienced by the subjects had gone into remission as a result of the natural history of the illness, with mainly negative and other residual symptoms remaining.
5. A large proportion of the cohort may have followed an episodic illness course with long intervals of quiescence of several years between the re-emergence of psychotic experiences. Thus, the 2-year period prior to the follow-up point may have failed to capture symptoms in subjects who would later experience relapses in terms of active psychotic symptoms.

Question A7

(i)   No. The findings would be of limited applicability in this case.

(ii)   This study cohort was assembled from individuals who had come into contact with psychiatric services. Those individuals who have a first episode of psychosis but do not engage with psychiatric services may potentially differ from the study cohort in a number of ways.

1. The family may have been more supportive than most where patients are engaged with psychiatry services, negating the need for more intensive mental health support.
2. It is also possible that Mr James's initial psychotic symptoms were more severe than many of the study subjects' and that this led him to be more resistant to contact with psychiatric services, perhaps as a result of paranoid ideation.
3. The choice of medication that the GP used may have differed from those generally employed by psychiatric services and might have influenced Mr James's symptoms and prognosis differently from those subjects in the study.
4. Mr James's initial symptoms may have been significantly less severe than those of the majority of the subjects in the study, allowing his family to manage him without the help of psychiatric services.

The lack of contact with psychiatric services may also have deprived Mr James of other interventions and treatments which potentially might have altered course and prognosis. Also, the family may have been more hostile in its attitude toward outside agencies than families that engage with mental health services, such as those in the study, and may have differed in other ways (e.g. they may have exhibited higher levels of expressed emotion).

Question BI

(i)   The standardised mortality rate calculates the ratio of the observed number of deaths in a specified group (in this case a group of individuals diagnosed with schizophrenia) to the expected number of deaths in the general population from which they are drawn (which would include both those with and without the condition of interest). The ratio is adjusted for age range and gender. The general population is usually that of a specified area, such as an electoral ward, or, as in this case, the catchment area of a district health authority. The units that SMR is expressed in can vary, but in this case it is expressed as a simple ratio.

(ii)

(a)   SMR is calculated by taking the number of observed deaths in the study population and dividing it by the number of expected deaths in the local general population from which they are drawn: i.e., SMR = observed deaths/expected deaths. Rearranging this simple equation: the number of observed deaths divided by the SMR will provide us with the value of the expected deaths. The SMR for male patients was 2.44 and the observed number of deaths in this group was 39. Thirty-nine divided by 2.44 gives us a value of 15.99. Rounding this figure up, the expected number of deaths in males of that age range from the general population in that particular catchment area would be 16.

(b)   Repeating the same calculations with the figures for females gives us: 30 (observed deaths) divided by 2.57 (SMR) is 11.67. Rounding up this means that 12 female deaths in general population for that age range would have been expected.

Question B2

(i)   No.

(ii)   Although the SMR for myocardial infarction is higher in women than in men (2.83 versus 1.42) this trend does not reach statistical significance as there is considerable overlap of the 95% confidence intervals for the SMR for this cause of death between the male and female groups. This indicates that we cannot be 95% confident that this observation would not have occurred by chance.

(iii)   Yes.

(iv)   The 95% confidence interval for the SMR for myocardial infarction in the female patients does not include or overlap a value of 1.0. This would indicate that we can be 95% confident that the difference between the observed and expected death rates is not due to chance and is thus statistically significant. The lower limit of 1.14 for the confidence interval would indicate that a woman with schizophrenia would be at least 14% more likely than a woman drawn from the general population to receive a verdict of death due to myocardial infarction.

Question B3

(i)   24 of the overall 69 deaths were unnatural (35%). This would appear to be a high proportion of the deaths that occurred in the patients with a diagnosis of schizophrenia. Although the majority did not receive a suicide verdict, the open verdict indicates that no other explanation was offered.

Even today suicide is a manner of death to which stigma is attached. This may be partly related to the fact that, in the past, people who died by suicide could not be buried in consecrated (holy) ground. Coroners are often reluctant to give suicide verdicts unless the circumstances clearly point to this cause of death, instead giving an open verdict. Thus, a suicide verdict is less likely in the absence of clear evidence of a planned attempt. The presence of a well-documented serious mental illness may also deter a coroner from giving a suicide verdict. Patients who are affected by schizophrenia may be less likely to leave evidence of a well-planned suicide attempt and thus receive a suicide verdict from the Coroner's Court.

Hence, it is possible that many of those unnatural deaths where an open verdict was given could actually have been the result of suicide. The use of suicide verdicts only could therefore significantly underestimate the SMR for this cause of death in patients with a diagnosis of schizophrenia. The inclusion of cases where an open verdict has been given in the case of an unnatural death may produce a more accurate reflection of the relative risk of suicide in this population.

(ii)
1.   A woman aged 15–44 years, with a diagnosis of schizophrenia, is statistically more likely to receive a suicide verdict following her death than a woman from the general population in that age range.

2.   A man aged 15–44 years, with a diagnosis of schizophrenia, is statistically more likely to receive a suicide verdict following his death than a man from the general population in that age range.

3.   A man aged over 44 years, with a diagnosis of schizophrenia, is not statistically significantly more likely to receive a suicide verdict following his death than a man drawn from the general population of over 44-year-olds. However, the presence of only one suicide verdict in this age and gender group means that we cannot be confident about this assertion on the basis of this study alone.

MRCPsych Part II Examination
Critical Review Paper
Spring 2000

Please read the instructions carefully before going further.

Instructions

1. This examination lasts for 90 minutes.
2. The paper has TWO questions, Question A and Question B. You must attempt ALL parts of BOTH questions.
3. A total of 100 marks has been allocated to the whole paper. Each part of each question is worth 10 marks. Therefore, Question A is worth 70 marks, and Question B is worth 30 marks.
4. In answering Question A, candidates may wish to glance briefly at the questions they are asked to answer (on pages 41–43 of the paper), before reading the details of the research (described on pages 38–40).
5. Candidates are advised to bring a calculator to the examination hall for this paper. Candidates are only permitted to take a noiseless, cordless, pocket-sized non-programmable calculator WITHOUT printout or graphic/word display facilities.
6. Please do not remove this Examination paper from the Examination Room.

Question A

Detecting mood disorders in general practice

Scenario

A local general practitioner asks you for advice about how to improve her ability to detect depression and anxiety in routine clinical practice. She and her partners have recently completed an audit of their management of patients whom they eventually refer to a psychiatrist for advice about depression. They have discovered that such patients have been frequent surgery attenders prior to referral, but with physical symptoms. She wonders if she and her partners have been missing depression in the earlier consultations, particularly in view of a recent paper she has found. She asks for your comments on the paper, which is:

Kessler, D., Lloyd, K., Lewis, G., *et al* (1999) Cross sectional study of symptom attribution and recognition of depression and anxiety in primary care. *British Medical Journal*, **318**, 436–439.

The paper

The paper evaluates the ability of general practitioners to identify anxiety and depression in attenders at routine surgeries. In this paper the diagnosis of depression or anxiety by the general practitioner is regarded as the test to be applied against the gold standard of the General Health Questionnaire (GHQ) score. The study also describes characteristics of the patients, which might have an influence on the judgement of general practitioners in detecting mood disorder.

Methodology

Setting

The study was undertaken in the UK, in a single urban general practice with eight partners, serving a population of 12 800 patients.

Sample

Consecutive attenders at surgery who were aged over 16 years.

Measures

1. The 12-item General Health Questionnaire (GHQ–12) was administered to all patients while they were waiting to see the doctor. A score of ⩾3 was used to identify people who were probable cases of depression or anxiety, although this information was not made available to the doctor at the time of the consultation. This score was chosen because, in an earlier study undertaken in primary care in the UK, it had been the optimal threshold for 'caseness' when compared with a more detailed psychiatric assessment.

2. At the same time, the patients completed the Symptom Interpretation Questionnaire (SIQ). In this instrument, patients are presented with a list of 13 common symptoms. They are asked to rate whether each symptom usually has a *somatic* cause, a *psychological* cause, or whether it is a feature of *normal* bodily function. The Questionnaire therefore yields three scores,

according to how many symptoms the patient attributes to each of these three causes. The three scores sum to 13. If the patient attributes the majority (seven or more) of symptoms to any one cause, he or she is described as predominantly *somatising, psychologising* or *normalising* in style, depending on which attribution is most used. If no attribution is used for the majority of symptoms, then the patient is described as having no predominant attributional style.

3. After the consultation, the general practitioners were asked to give each patient a psychiatric diagnosis if appropriate, and to say whether any anxiety or depression was new or already known.

Results

1. Of 355 consecutive attenders, 26 (7%) refused to participate and 24 (6.8%) returned incomplete questionnaires. In the remaining 305, there were 225 women and 80 men. The average age of the patients was 44 years (range 16–90). Men were slightly older than women (49 years *v.* 42 years).
2. The GHQ–12 identified 157 (52%) people as cases using the cut-off $\geqslant 3$.
3. The general practitioners diagnosed 71 (24%) people as cases of anxiety, depression or both.
4. Results on the SIQ showed that 145 (48%) patients were predominantly 'normalisers', 71 (23%) were predominantly 'psychologisers', and only 16 (5%) were predominantly 'somatisers', 72 (24%) had no predominant attributional style.
5. Other results are shown in Tables A1 and A2.

Table A1. Ability of general practitioners (GPs) to identify cases of depression or anxiety (as defined by GHQ–12 score)

	GHQ–12 defined case	GHQ–12 defined non-case	Total
GP diagnosed case	57	14	71
GP diagnosed non-case	100	134	234
Total	157	148	305

Table A2. Detection by general practitioner of anxiety and depression in 305 patients according to style of symptom attribution

	Predominant attribution type (score 7 or more)			
	Psychologising	Normalising	Somatising	No predominant score
Total sample				
Number of patients	71	146	16	72
Number of women (%)	61 (86)	99 (68)	9 (56)	56 (78)
Mean age (years)	43.4	40.4	58.6	48.8
Number (%)	55 (77)	54 (37)	6 (38)	42 (58)
GHQ cases				
Number not detected*	21	46	5	29
Percentage not detected	38	85	83	69
95% CI**	25 to 52	73 to 93	36 to 100	53 to 82

*'Not detected', patients classified as cases according to the GHQ–12 but not diagnosed as such by the general practitioner.

**95% CI, 95% confidence interval of percentage of GHQ cases not detected.

Question B

Early life family disadvantages and major depression in adulthood

Table B1 has been modified from:

Sadowski, H., Ugarte, B., Kolvin, I., *et al* (1999) Early life family disadvantages and major depression in adulthood. *British Journal of Psychiatry*, **174**, 112–120.

Table B1 reports results from a study which followed a cohort of children into adult life. The main aim of the study was to determine whether disadvantages in early family life were associated with major depression later in adulthood. From the original cohort ($n=781$) a sample was taken ($n=301$) and assessed at 33 years of age. The presence of major depression in the year before assessment was the main outcome. For the analysis, the sample was divided into those who had experienced 'multiple disadvantage' in childhood, and those who had not.

Table B1. One-year prevalence of major depressive disorder at 33 years of age in relation to 'multiple disadvantage' experienced in the first 5 years of life

	No multiple disadvantage group	Multiple disadvantage group	Odds ratio	95% CI*
Sample population				
Total	16/223 (7.2%)	11/39 (28.2%)	5.1	2.1 to 12.0
Females	12/108 (11.1%)	7/22 (31.8%)	3.7	1.3 to 11.0
Males	4/115 (3.5%)	4/17 (23.5%)	8.5	1.9 to 38.3

*95% CI, 95% confidence interval of odds ratio.

Question A

NOTE: Each question is worth 10 marks. There are a total of 100 marks for the whole paper, 70 marks for Question A and 30 marks for Question B.

Question AI

In this paper, it is assumed that the GHQ–12 is a valid means of identifying depression and anxiety. Define what is meant by the validity of a measure.

[2 marks]

Briefly describe *two* types of validity of such instruments.

[6 marks]

When employing a standard measure of psychiatric illness to validate the GHQ what is the main requirement of subject samples used in such investigations?

[2 marks]

Question A2

The authors use a threshold score of 3 on the GHQ–12 for defining psychiatric disorder, because this was the optimal cut-off for defining 'caseness' when the GHQ–12 was compared with more detailed psychiatric assessment in a different study. Define the optimal threshold for any diagnostic test.

[3 marks]

Give *two* reasons why it may be difficult to set the optimal threshold score of the GHQ and psychiatric assessment in this study.

[4 marks]

How would a receiver operator curve (ROC) assist in this exercise?

[3 marks]

Question A3

The results include the reported sensitivity and specificity of the general practitioners' diagnoses. Define sensitivity and specificity.

[2 + 2 marks]

Calculate the sensitivity and specificity of the diagnostic categories given by the general practitioners from the data described in Table A1.

[2 + 2 marks]

From these results, if a general practitioner makes the diagnosis of anxiety or depression, how confident can you be that the patient concerned will be a GHQ-defined case?

[2 marks]

Question A4

What is the *positive predictive value* of a test?

[3 marks]

Use the data in Table A1 to calculate the positive predictive value of a general practitioner diagnosis of depression or anxiety in identifying GHQ-defined cases.

[3 marks]

Explain whether or not you expect the positive predictive value to change, and in what direction, if the same study was carried out using patients in a general medical ward.

[4 marks]

Question A5

Table A2 shows the relation between scores on the symptom attribution questionnaire, the rate of GHQ caseness, and the rate of non-detection of GHQ cases by the general practitioner. Give *five* main findings from the results shown in the table, with reference to differences between the three attributional style groups.

[2 marks for each finding, up to a maximum of 10 marks]

Question A6

The last rows of Table A2 present data showing the proportion of GHQ cases which were not detected by general practitioners. Associated with each rate is a 95% confidence interval. Define the 95% confidence interval.

[3 marks]

Explain what it means.

[4 marks]

Why is the confidence interval for the non-detection of patients with a somatising attributional style wider than for the patients with a normalising style when the percentage of patients in each group is almost identical?

[3 marks]

Question A7

Your general practitioner colleague's original question was about patients who finally are referred to a psychiatrist, querying whether initial presentation with physical symptoms might lead to the general practitioners initially missing a diagnosis of depression. How far does this paper assist her in proving or disproving her hypothesis that some depressed patients are not diagnosed because they present with physical symptoms?

[1 mark]

Explain your reasoning.

[2 marks]

Does the paper help her in determining which patients she should refer to the psychiatrists?

[1 mark]

Explain your conclusions.

[3 marks]

How accurate is the diagnosis of depression and anxiety made according to the threshold score of $\geqslant 3$ on the GHQ?

[1 mark]

Indicate your reasoning.

[2 marks]

Question B

Question BI

The rate for major depression is expressed as a one-year prevalence. What type of prevalence is this called?

[3 marks]

What other type of prevalence is there?

[3 marks]

Indicate whether this alternative method of describing prevalence is likely to lead to a smaller or greater number of cases of depression. Explain your reasoning.

[4 marks]

Question B2

If the *odds* of an event happening are 1 in 9, what would be the *rate* or *frequency* of that event?

[3 marks]

Table BI expresses the difference between the two groups as an odds ratio. Explain exactly what is meant by the odds ratio of 5.1 in Table BI.

[4 marks]

If the odds ratio was 1.0 in any group of the sample population what would this mean?

[3 marks]

Question B3

Give *four* main findings shown in Table BI with particular relevance to the meaning of the odds ratios and their confidence intervals. Include in these the differences between men and women shown in the table, indicating whether these are likely to be significant.

[10 marks]

Model answers by Ayla Khan

Question Al

(i)   Validity of a measure is used to describe whether it measures what it purports to measure.

(ii)   Concurrent validity – compares whether the test maintains validity compared with an external existing valid test at the same time.

Cross validity – determines whether the test maintains validity if it is applied to another sample/setting.

(iii)   The main requirement is that the data are obtained from patients similar to those used in the GHQ.

Question A2

(i)   Optimal threshold is the level at which false negatives and positives are at their minimum level: or, at the point where sensitivity and specificity are at their maximum or optimum level.

(ii) The threshold score for caseness on the GHQ-12 used in the paper was taken from an earlier study. It may not be generalisable to other populations, because of possible differences in gender, ethnicity, social class, etc. Furthermore, the distribution of GHQ scores may have changed since the threshold score was set.

The gold standard for diagnosis in the study is the GHQ, but this is a screening test for psychiatric disorder, not a diagnostic measure. The GP's diagnosis is the test applied against this gold standard. Setting the optimal threshold score for the GHQ involves trading off false positive and false negative rates. Here, the GPs do not want to miss patients with depression, so a low cut-off score (which will reduce false negatives) is better.

(iii)   A receiver operator curve could be generated to produce a graph at different cut-offs on the GHQ for caseness. The knee or shoulder of the curve chooses the cut-off that optimises both sensitivity and specificity.

Question A3

(i)   Sensitivity – proportion of people who have the disorder who are correctly identified as positive by the test.

Specificity – proportion of people who do not have the disorder who are correctly identified as negative by the test.

(ii)   Sensitivity $= 57/157 = 36.3\%$

Specificity $= 134/148 = 90.5\%$

(iii)   One can be only 36% confident that the patient concerned is a GHQ-defined case.

Question A4

(i)   Positive predictive value of a test is defined as the proportion of people with a positive test who have the disorder (true positives).

(ii)   PPV is $57/71 = 80.3\%$

(iii)   One would expect the PPV to change if the test was carried out on a medical ward. It would decrease, as the prevalence of psychiatric cases would be less. PPV decreases as prevalence of disorder decreases.

Question A5

(i)   86% of the psychologising group are women, compared with 68% and 56% in the normalising and somatising groups respectively.

Mean age of somatising group is 58.6 years; i.e. much older than the psychologising and normalising groups, which were 43.4 and 40.4 years respectively.

Of the GHQ cases, high percentages of the normalisers and somatisers (85% and 83%) were not detected as cases, compared with only 38% of psychologisers not detected.

77% of psychologisers were detected as GHQ cases, compared with only 37% and 38% of normalising and somatising groups respectively.

Of the GHQ cases, the psychologisers and normalisers have a narrow confidence interval, compared with the somatisers, who have a wide confidence interval.

Question A6

(i)   The 95% confidence interval (CI) is a statistical term to define the range within which one can be 95% confident that the true value lies.

(ii)   It means that in a range of, e.g. 25–52, one can be 95% certain/confident that the actual/true value lies within this range. There is therefore a 5% chance the true value may lie outside this range.

(iii)   The CI for non-detection of somatisers is wider than that for normalisers because the total number of people in this group is much fewer. A larger sample size is much more likely to yield true results.

Question A7

(i)   The paper proves the hypothesis that some depressed patients are missed because they present with physical symptoms.

(ii)   It shows that GPs in the study miss a proportion of true cases as defined by a cut-off score on the GHQ (83% of somatisers were missed).

(iii)   Yes, somewhat.

(iv)   The paper suggests that GPs should be more aware that some patients, particularly those with normalising and somatising attributional styles, often get missed diagnostically. These could then be further screened and referred on to psychiatrists.

(v)   The diagnosis made according to a GHQ score ⩾3 is fairly accurate.

(vi)   This is because it has been tested on a previous sample based in primary care, i.e. a similar setting. This showed that a score ⩾3 yielded the optimum threshold for caseness.

Question B1

(i)   Period prevalence is the prevalence of a disorder over a given period of time.

(ii)   Point prevalence is the prevalence of a disorder at a given point in time.

(iii)   Point prevalence would lead to a smaller number of cases of depression, as it is only taken at a specific time point, rather than over a period of time.

Question B2

(i)   If the odds of an event are 1:9, the rate or frequency would be 1/10 (10%).

(ii)   The odds ratio (OR) is the ratio of the odds, i.e. it compares the odds of outcomes in 2 different groups. In this case, the odds ratio of 5.1 means that those people with multiple disadvantage (MD) in early family life are 5.1 times more likely to have major depression in adulthood than those with no multiple disadvantage (NMD).

(iii)   If the OR is 1.0 this means that there is no difference in the odds of the outcome occurring in the 2 groups that are being compared; i.e. there is no effect.

Question B3

Males are 8.5 times more likely to have depression if MD than NMD. This has a wide confidence interval (CI).

Females are 3.7 times more likely to have depression if MD than if NMD. This has a narrow CI.

One is 5.1 times more likely to have depression if MD than if NMD. This has a narrow CI.

All the CIs for the OR indicated in the study are significant, as none of them cross 1.

MRCPsych Part II Examination
Critical Review Paper
Autumn 2000

Please read the instructions carefully before going further.

Instructions

1. This examination lasts for 90 minutes.
2. The paper has TWO questions, Question A and Question B. You must attempt ALL parts of BOTH questions.
3. A total of 100 marks has been allocated to the whole paper. Each part of each question is worth 10 marks. Therefore, Question A is worth 70 marks, and Question B is worth 30 marks.
4. In answering Question A, candidates may wish to glance briefly at the questions they are asked to answer (on pages 52–54 of the paper), before reading the details of the research (described on pages 48–50).
5. Candidates are advised to bring a calculator to the examination hall for this paper. Candidates are only permitted to take a noiseless, cordless, pocket-sized non-programmable calculator WITHOUT printout or graphic/word display facilities.
6. Please do not remove this Examination paper from the Examination Room.

Question A

Treatment of acute mania

Scenario

AB is a 25-year-old woman with bipolar affective disorder, who has just been admitted under the Mental Health Act with a manic episode. She has had two affective episodes in the last two years, the first depressive and the second manic. She has been on lithium since the last manic episode from which she recovered nine months ago. Plasma lithium levels have been in the range of 0.8–1.0 mmol/l.

You recently read a review, which suggested that lithium is ineffective, or poorly tolerated in at least one third of treated patients. You have heard that sodium valproate may be helpful in the treatment of mania.

You perform a literature search and find the following recent paper.

Bowden CL, Brugger AM, Swann AC, *et al*: Efficacy of Divalproex vs Lithium and Placebo in the Treatment of Mania. *JAMA*, 1994; 271, No 12, 918–924.

The methods and results are summarised below.

The paper

This paper describes a study comparing the effectiveness of divalproex (a preparation of sodium valproate and valproic acid) with that of (a) lithium and (b) placebo in patients with acute mania.

Methods

This is a double-blind, multicentre, randomised controlled trial of divalproex v. lithium v. placebo given in flexible dosage for 21 days, after a washout period to eliminate other drugs.

Inclusion criteria

- RDC diagnosis of acute mania
- Aged between 18–65 years
- Mania Rating Scale (MRS) score of at least 14 prior to randomisation. The MRS is a subscale of the Schedule for Affective Disorders and Schizophrenia and rates elevated mood, less need for sleep, excessive energy, excessive activity, grandiosity, irritability, motor hyperactivity, accelerated speech, racing thoughts, and poor judgement. It is a well-validated measure of severity of mania.

Exclusion criteria

- A history of severe side effects from lithium
- Prior treatment with divalproex
- CNS/neuromuscular disease; other uncontrolled medical illness or pregnancy
- Substance abuse
- Concomitant treatment with medication that would confound the results.

Recovery Criterion

A reduction in MRS score of at least 50% from its baseline value.

Termination criteria

Patients left the study early if they:
- Required extra psychoactive medications not specified in the protocol
- Developed severe depression
- Had an increase of greater than 30% in their MRS score
- Met the recovery criterion (see above) and, in addition, showed no MRS item score above 2 *and* had a Global Assessment Scale score higher than 70.

Randomisation

Patients were assigned by block randomisation to divalproex, lithium or placebo in a 2:1:2 ratio. A separate randomisation schedule was generated for each centre prior to the start of the study. The allocation list was concealed from clinicians and patients. Centres were sent patient numbers in blocks of 10; unknown to the investigators, treatment group assignments were randomised in blocks of 5 within each set of ten numbers.

Procedure

Patients who were already on psychoactive drugs when recruited had a washout period equivalent to either 3 days or 5 half-lives of the longest-acting psychoactive drug they had been taking, whichever was the longer.

Both patients and clinicians remained blind to the treatment allocation following randomisation. Comparable adjustments were made in the dosages of divalproex, lithium and placebo according to protocol-specified dosing schedules, which were set primarily according to the plasma levels of the drugs. These adjustments were made by a clinician who knew the group to which the patient had been assigned, but without the knowledge of the other participants. For divalproex and lithium, dosages were adjusted (as permitted by patient tolerance of the drug) to reach pre-defined plasma levels.

The trial lasted 21 days from the start of the trial medication. The MRS and the Global Assessment Scale were administered to all patients on days 1, 5, 10, 15 and 21.

Other drugs

Neuroleptic drugs were not allowed and any patient who required these drugs for clinical reasons was withdrawn from the study. The use of chloral hydrate or lorazepam was allowed as needed to control agitation, irritability, restlessness, insomnia and hostility. The details of adjunctive drugs actually used within each treatment group were not reported.

Statistical analysis

All randomised patients were included in the analysis and they were analysed according to the treatment group to which they were initially assigned. If a patient dropped out of the study, the last available MRS observation was used for the analysis. Continuous variables were compared by the overall F test of one-way analysis of variance (ANOVA) and categorical variables by Fisher's Exact Test.

Results

Baseline characteristics

A total of 179 patients were randomised. Table AI shows the characteristics of the three groups of patients before treatment.

89% of patients had experienced prior manic episodes, a median period of 13.5 years had elapsed since the first manic episode, and a median time of 9.5 months had elapsed since the last manic episode. 71% had experienced major depressive episodes. A median period of 15.0 years had elapsed since the first depressive episode, and a median time of 12.5 months since the last depressive episode. 88% had previously been admitted to a psychiatric hospital.

The three groups had comparable prior treatment for the current episode of mania prior to entry into the study.

Main results

Clinical response (at least a 50% reduction from the baseline MRS score) occurred in 48% of the divalproex group, 49% of the lithium group and 25% of the placebo group.

The response rates in the two drug-treated groups were significantly greater than the improvement observed in the placebo group ($p=0.004$ for divalproex and $p=0.025$ for lithium).

Table AI. **Characteristics of the three groups of patients before treatment**

	Treatment group		
Characteristic	Divalproex	Lithium	Placebo
Number of patients	69	36	74
Age: years (mean +/− SD)	40.4 +/−12.8	39.1 +/−11.2	39.0 +/−10.0
Sex: % male/female	52:48	72:28	57:43
Race: % white:black:other	73:17:10	66:17:17	72:19:9
Length of illness, years (mean +/− SD)	18.0 +/−12.4	16.1 +/−11.0	18.0 +/−10.4
Four or more bipolar episodes per year in the past 2 years*			
Any mood disorder: number (%)	11 (19)	1 (4)	6 (10)
Mania only: number (%)**	8 (14)†	0	0
Prior lithium treatment, No. (%)	54 (78)	31 (86)	61 (82)
Effective, tolerated ***	22 (41)	16 (52)	19 (31)
Effective, not tolerated ***	7 (13)	0	6 (10)
Ineffective, tolerated ***	19 (35)	11 (35)	31 (51)
Ineffective, not tolerated ***	6 (11)	4 (13)	5 (8)

*Four or more bipolar episodes per year for 2 years indicates rapid cycling.

**Percentages based on total number of patients with available histories in each group.

***Percentages based on numbers of patients who took lithium previously.

†Patients in the divalproex group had a significantly higher incidence of manic episodes than those in the other two groups ($p<0.05$).

Question B

Lithium discontinuation during early pregnancy

Figure I is taken from a recently published paper: Viguera AC *et al*: Risk of recurrence of bipolar disorder in pregnant and non-pregnant women after discontinuing lithium maintenance. *American Journal of Psychiatry* 2000; 157: 179–184.

The authors retrospectively studied recurrence rates and survival to relapse in 101 women with DSM–IV bipolar disorder over a 64-week follow-up period after discontinuing lithium. Forty two of the women were recruited at the onset of pregnancy and followed up through the post-partum period. They had all discontinued lithium treatment within six weeks of conception. Fifty-nine age-matched non-pregnant control patients were followed up for equivalent periods (weeks 1–40 and 41–64).

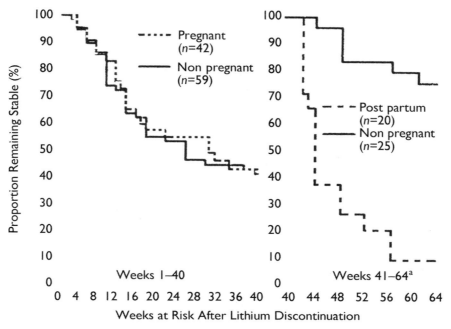

Figure 1.

Question A

NOTE: Each question is worth 10 marks. There are a total of 100 marks for the whole paper, 70 marks for Question A and 30 marks for Question B.

Question A1

List *five* features of the design of this study which should help to minimise bias favouring one treatment over another. For each feature you list, explain briefly how it might reduce bias.

[1 mark for each feature and 1 for each explanation]

Question A2

List *five* potential or actual weaknesses of the study. For each point you list, explain how it might affect the outcome of the study.

[1 mark for each feature and 1 for each explanation]

Question A3

(a) If the main objective of the study was to evaluate the efficacy of divalproex, why was a lithium arm included in this study? (Refer to the data in Table A1 as appropriate.)

[5 marks]

(b) If a lithium arm is included, why is a placebo arm required?

[5 marks]

Question A4

(a) What advantage is there to having the patients randomised in blocks?

[4 marks]

(b) Why in this study were randomisation blocks of 5 used, rather than the more common 4?

[3 marks]

(c) What is the significance of the researchers and clinicians being unaware that patients had been allocated in blocks of 5?

[3 marks]

Question A5

With regard to those patients showing the agreed defined clinical response:

(a)   What is the absolute benefit of divalproex compared with placebo?

[2 marks]

(b)   What is the relative difference in the proportion of patients responding on divalproex compared with those receiving placebo (the Relative Benefit Increase)?

[2 marks]

(c)   Calculate the number needed to treat (NNT) for divalproex compared with placebo.

[2 marks]

(d)   How do you interpret this value?

[4 marks]

Question A6

Considering the results of the study:

(a)   What does this study suggest about the anti-manic efficacy of lithium?

[I mark]

(b)   How is your conclusion affected, if at all, by the data in Table AI on patients' prior treatment with lithium?

[3 marks]

(c)   Although the effect of lithium was comparable with the effect of divalproex, certain comparisons of lithium with placebo in Table AI did not reach significance. Why not?

[2 marks]

(d)   What is the importance of the statistically significant finding in Table AI, that patients in the divalproex group were more likely than those assigned to the other two groups to have a history of 4 or more manic episodes annually in the preceding 2 years?

[4 marks]

Question A7

(a)   How applicable are the results of the study to your patient?

[I mark]

(b)   Justify your answer with reference to the information in the summary.

[2 marks]

(c)   For patient AB, give one advantage for administration of divalproex and one advantage for administration of lithium.

[2 marks for each]

(d)   Which drug is your preferred choice?

[I mark]

(e)   Give *two* further reasons to justify your preferred choice of drug.

[I mark for each point made, to a total of 2]

Question B

Question BI

Describe *five* important features that are shown in Figure I.

[2 marks for each relevant point]

Question B2

The authors discuss the possibility that confounding might bias their results.

(a)   What does the term *confounder* mean?

[4 marks]

(b)   Give *two* examples of possible confounders in this study.

[2 marks]

(c) Explain how they might be expected to influence the observed outcome.

[4 marks]

Question B3

(a) Describe the *two* main conclusions that you draw from the graph presented.

[2 marks for each explanation, up to a maximum of 4]

(b) Give *three* recommendations about how these conclusions would inform clinical practice.

[2 marks for each up to a maximum of 6]

Model answers by Danny H. Sullivan

Question AI

1.   The use of RDC criteria – reduces selection bias by ensuring that all subjects have a validated diagnosis which satisfies agreed symptom criteria.

2.   Applying the Mania Rating Scale – reduces selection bias by ensuring that all subjects exhibit at least a certain amount of disease severity.

3.   Blinding – prevents clinicians from favouring those they might know are in the treatment group. Differential treatment of one group might lead to performance bias.

4.   Randomisation with allocation concealment – systematic allocation of patients to random groups prevents researchers from conscious or unconscious allocation to a preferred treatment group, for instance in those they believe would benefit from one treatment above another.

5.   Intention-to-treat analysis – reduces the likelihood that non-responders are excluded from study results, and thus the study demonstrates a benefit in excess of its actual effects, otherwise known as attrition bias.

Question A2

1.   The exclusion criteria prevent many actual patients from enrolment; a sample of adult age, tolerant of lithium, and not misusing substances, is not representative of real world subjects. They may respond better than real subjects and thus the results might be more significant than in a clinical population.

2.   An endpoint of 50% reduction in the score on the Mania Rating Scale might not correlate with a clinically significant reduction in symptoms. Subjects with very high scores at the commencement of the study may remain quite manic.

3.   Despite a washout period, the effects of previous treatment may interfere with the experimental treatment. For instance, those recently ceasing lithium may be at increased risk of relapse or of rebound mania. This may result in a slower response for the lithium arm.

4.   Adjunctive medications such as lorazepam and chloral hydrate may confound the beneficial effects of medication: thus, should a trial treatment be ineffective, this might be masked by increasing benzodiazepine use in that group. Use of adjunctive drugs was not reported and therefore it is uncertain whether there were significant differences in their use between the study arms.

5.   A study protocol not involving the use of antipsychotic medications differs markedly from actual clinical practice. Although the protocol excludes antipsychotic medications, to prevent confounding, this may result in the study lacking generalisability to routine clinical situations.

Question A3

(a)
1.   Lithium is included because it is the gold standard treatment for acute mania, with a substantial evidence base for use.

2.   Comparison with lithium enables clear validation of results against an existing benchmark.

3.   It may be unethical to deny treatment to people with acute mania, thus limiting the use of trial drugs against placebo alone.

4.   Comparison with lithium enables direct comparison rather than having to rely on a crossover design, which is more expensive, challenging to conduct and lengthier.

5.   To gain marketing approval for a specific indication, it is usually necessary to demonstrate at least equal efficacy with an existing treatment for the condition.

(b)   A placebo arm demonstrates that improvement is due to active treatment rather than non-study variables. Placebo effects might induce improvement, as might variables not studied in this trial, such as admission to hospital and management in an intensive care unit. Other variables which might account for improvement include the Hawthorne effect, extra attention paid to subjects by researchers, or the use of adjunctive medication. A placebo arm allows clear demonstration that the treatment itself is effective, rather than contingencies.

Question A4

(a)   Block randomisation is useful in smaller trials to maintain balance between treatment arms. At any time, there will be approximately equal numbers in treatment arms. Serial allocation, although simpler, is open to unblinding as the pattern becomes apparent; and simple randomisation might lead to unbalanced allocation to groups.

(b)   Blocks of 5 are effective for the study design of 2:1:2 and permit allocation of appropriate numbers to each arm. Using blocks which are a multiple of the number of trial groups is logical.

(c)   If researchers and clinicians are unaware that block randomised patients were allocated in groups of 5, this further reduces the chance for bias to intrude into allocation to study arms. Centralised randomisation improves allocation concealment, as does a protocol which is less likely to be perceived or predicted by investigators.

Question A5

(a)   Absolute benefit+absolute benefit increase (ABI):
ABI=Experimental event rate (EER)−Control event rate (CER)
$$=48\%-25\%$$
$$=23\%$$

(b)   Relative benefit increase (RBI):
RBI=(EER−CER)/CER
$$=23\%/25\%$$
$$=92\%$$

(c)   Number need to treat:
NNT=1/ABI
$$=1/.23$$
$$=4.35$$
$$\geqslant 5$$

(d)   An NNT of 5 refers to the number of patients required to be treated with divalproex for one additional treatment success. Generally, an NNT less than 10 indicates that a treatment is clinically significant. Obviously, the nature of the outcome, its application in large treatment groups, or expense may modify the NNT regarded as clinically significant.

Question A6

(a)   This study suggests that lithium, with a response rate of 49%, is effective for the acute treatment of mania.

(b)   Although effective as a treatment, 28 out of 146 patients previously treated with lithium were unable to tolerate it. In addition, almost all of the patients who were rapid-cycling fell into the divalproex group, which may have skewed results in favour of lithium.

(c)   Some comparisons of lithium and placebo may not have reached significance because the lithium group was small in number. Unless a large number of subjects were used, a small or moderate difference between small groups may not achieve significance.

(d)   It is important to note that the divalproex group contained a significantly higher number of subjects with four or manic episodes in the preceding two years. These rapid-cycling patients tend to have a poorer response to lithium. Thus, their presence in the divalproex group, despite chance allocation, may lead to skewed results through selection bias. It would be important to analyse the data both with and without these patients to ensure that their presence did not alter results.

Question A7

(a)   The patient, a 25-year-old woman, is within the study parameters demographically, and her illness qualifies for study inclusion. Thus, the study results may be applied to her.

(b)   The patient would have qualified for enrolment because of age and gender; not only do her number of illnesses, diagnosis and prior treatment conform to enrolment, but there are no factors suggesting that she would not be eligible for recruitment. Thus, the results of the study are generalisable to our patient.

(c)   Lithium is clearly tolerated by patient AB, judging by her persistent treatment with it.
Divalproex may cause fewer side effects and thus reduce withdrawal from the treatment.

(d)   I would prefer divalproex, because of the failure of lithium in this patient to prevent both depressive and manic episodes at high therapeutic plasma levels, and its apparent equivalent efficacy in the treatment of acute manic episodes.

(e)   Divalproex may offer less risk of hypothyroidism or renal impairment in the longer term, should it be used as prophylaxis. It is generally well tolerated and has side-effects perceived by many patients as less troublesome than those of lithium. It often has more rapid onset of action compared with lithium.

Question B1

1.   The Kaplan–Meier survival curve shows that there is no difference in bipolar disorder relapse rates between pregnant and non-pregnant women who discontinue lithium.

2.   Pregnancy does not appear to be protective against relapse in women who discontinue lithium.

3.   There was a marked increase in relapse rates in the post-partum period compared with the non-pregnant group.

4.   The median survival to relapse is four weeks post-partum.

5.   Almost all women who discontinue lithium relapse in the post-partum six months.

Question B2

(a)   A confounder is a variable which may affect study outcome. It is a variable which is associated with the exposure and may predict the outcome of interest. Thus, a confounder may produce a false association between exposure and outcome, or conceal a true association. It should not be on the direct causal pathway and it must differ between the comparison groups. In providing an alternative explanation for study results, a confounder may render results invalid if an attempt is not made to exclude or control for confounding variables.

(b)   The effects of lithium cessation may act as confounders in this study, particularly if there is a differential effect in pregnancy. Stressors in the post-partum period, such as sleep deprivation or marital discord, may independently contribute to relapse when compared with non-pregnant women and thus act as confounders.

(c)   Lithium discontinuation may precipitate relapse, particularly if rapid. Thus, pregnancy may be protective against relapse, but the effect could be concealed by rapid discontinuation precipitating relapse in the pregnant group.
If stressors disproportionately affect the post-partum group, they may result in relapse. The non-pregnant group might then appear less likely to relapse, owing to a relative dearth of stressors, but this might not be attributable to lithium discontinuation.

Question B3

(a)   Over 50% of women will relapse within 6 months following discontinuation. Thus, it is not necessarily safe for women to cease lithium on learning of pregnancy.
The post-partum period poses an extremely high risk of relapse. Women who choose to remain off lithium should be closely monitored for signs of relapse.

(b)   These conclusions suggest that:

1.   Women should be advised of the risks of discontinuing lithium, and a risk–benefit analysis should inform pregnant women taking lithium of whether discontinuation is warranted, balancing a hypothetical increase in foetal malformations with the consequences of relapse.
2.   For those who discontinue lithium, medication should be reinstated soon after delivery to reduce the risk of subsequent and rapid relapse. Breastfeeding is contraindicated in this population.
3.   Those who determine that they will not recommence lithium should be monitored closely for signs of relapse, and treatment reinstated as soon as necessary to reduce disruption to mother–infant interactions.

MRCPsych Part II Examination
Critical Review Paper
Spring 2001

Please read the instructions carefully before going further.

Instructions

1. This examination lasts for 90 minutes.
2. The paper has TWO questions, Question A and Question B. You must attempt ALL parts of BOTH questions.
3. A total of 100 marks has been allocated to the whole paper. Each part of each question is worth 10 marks. Therefore, Question A is worth 70 marks, and Question B is worth 30 marks.
4. In answering Question A, candidates may wish to glance briefly at the questions they are asked to answer (on pages 63–65 of the paper), before reading the details of the research (described on pages 60–63).
5. Candidates are advised to bring a calculator to the examination hall for this paper. Candidates are only permitted to take a noiseless, cordless, pocket-sized non-programmable calculator WITHOUT printout or graphic/word display facilities.
6. Please do not remove this Examination paper from the Examination Room.

Question A

Strategies for suicide prevention

Scenario

You are contacted by your local Director of Public Health, who wishes to discuss with you a paper about which she has been told. She understands that the paper indicates that a high proportion of people who have committed suicide turn out to have been taking psychotropic medication. Based on this, she poses two specific questions. First, could information from the paper be used in everyday clinical practice to help to identify psychiatric patients at high risk of suicide? The Director of Public Health is also keen to meet local targets for reduction in suicide rates, and her second question is − might data from the paper support an intervention targeting people attending the psychiatric outpatient clinic as a means of meeting the target of reducing suicide rates?

Summary of the paper

The paper concerned is:

Boardman AP, Grimbaldeston AH, Handley C, Jones PW, Willmott S. The North Staffordshire suicide study: a case-control study of suicide in one health district. *Psychological Medicine* 1999; 29: 27–33.

The paper describes a project aiming to identify sociodemographic and clinical risk factors for death from suicide and undetermined injury in residents in the catchment area of a single health authority.

The setting of the research project

The health authority concerned covers an area of 340 square miles and has a population of approximately 471,000, with approximately four-fifths of the population living in urban areas, and the remainder in a very rural area. A single mental health service covers the whole catchment area of North Staffordshire. The rate of suicide and undetermined injury in the area, as well as trends over time, are in line with national data.

Identification of cases

Residents of the district dying from suicide (ICD-9 E95-959) or undetermined injury (ICD-9 E980-989) over the 5-year period 1 January 1991 to 31 December 1995 were identified from Office of Population Census and Surveys (OPCS) Regional Death Tapes. These OPCS data are anonymised, but individuals were identified by matching dates of birth and death and postcode from the OPCS data with records from the Coroner's Inquest Register and death registration returns to the Department of Public Health Medicine.

Cases were included if the individuals had been resident in North Staffordshire at the time of death, even if death occurred outside the district. Any individuals not resident in North Staffordshire at the time of death were excluded. Cases were also excluded if according to the Coroner's records (scrutinised by members of the research team) the final verdict was of homicide or of reckless driving, or if the circumstances of death appeared unrelated to self-harm and the Coroner had investigated and dismissed the possibility of suicide.

Identification of controls

These were also gathered from cases reported to the Coroner. From the Coroner's records, age and sex matched individuals dying during the same 5-year period for reasons other than those identifying cases (as above) were obtained.

Data collection

Three sources of information were used.

(a) Coroner's inquest records (including witness statements, medical and post mortem reports, other legal documents, suicide notes, photographs etc).
(b) General practitioner records (following a patient's death, his/her records return to the Family Health Services Authority, and it was from here that the records were sought).
(c) Hospital records, including medical records and records from the two catchment area psychiatric hospitals and associated satellite clinics (which included mental health centres and day hospitals) plus the hospital computer database.

Psychiatric diagnoses were identified in the Coroner's records, and then confirmed with reference to medical or therapeutic evidence in the inquest file and/or the case-notes. The clinical members of the research team agreed final diagnoses (according to ICD-10). Multiple diagnoses were allowed.

Analysis

All predictors were transformed to binary variables, to simplify analysis. Individual predictors were tested by comparing cases and controls in a pairwise fashion using McNemar's Test.

Results

Of the 212 cases, 167 were male (79%, male:female ratio=3.7:1). The median age was 43 years (range 14–89 years). 58% of the men and 44% of the women were aged under 45 years (Chi square=2.67; df=1; p=0.103). In men, the commonest cause of death was by hanging (32%) or by motor vehicle exhaust (26%). In women, the commonest cause of death was overdose of medication (47%). Among the suicide cases, 43% had left a note.

Comparisons of cases and matched controls on the univariate predictor variables are shown in Table A1 (sociodemographic and clinical factors including life events and difficulties) and Table A2 (health service contact and prescribed medication).

Table A1   Comparison of cases and matched controls – sociodemographic and clinical variables, life events and difficulties

Variable	No of cases (N=212)	No of controls (N=212)	Odds ratio	95% CI of OR**
Sociodemographic				
Living alone	83	38	2.8*	1.7–4.6
Single (no known relationship)	37	57	0.5*	0.3–0.9
Married	66	88	0.6*	0.4–1.0
Separated	43	8	5.9*	2.6–15.5
Divorced	13	18	0.8	0.3–1.7
Widowed	25	15	2.1	0.9–5.3
Unemployed	42	21	2.8*	1.4–5.9
Retired	13	18	0.7	0.3–1.6
Life events and difficulties				
Recent bereavement	61	28	2.7*	1.6–4.7
Recent separation	85	17	7.2*	3.8–15.0
Financial difficulties	41	6	6.8*	2.9–19.7
Relationship difficulties	107	28	8.2*	4.4–17.0
Work stress	26	0	*#	#
Clinical variables				
Any confirmed psychiatric diagnosis	151	94	3.5*	2.2–5.8
Depression only	79	43	2.8*	1.7–4.9
Bipolar affective disorder	3	1	3.0	0.2–158
Schizophrenia	7	3	2.3	0.5–14.0
Alcohol abuse	40	34	1.2	0.7–2.1
Drug abuse	11	10	1.1	0.4–2.9
Personality disorder	28	16	1.9	1.0–4.1
Past contact with psychiatric services	88	24	5.3*	3.0–9.9
Past history of deliberate self-harm	110	27	11.5*	5.6–27.4

*P < 0.05 (McNemar Test); ** 95% Confidence Interval of Odds Ratio; # Unable to calculate due to missing cells

Table A2   Comparison of cases and matched controls — health service contacts and medication prescribed before death

Variable	No of cases (N = 212)	No of controls (N = 212)	Odds ratio	95% CI of OR**
Health service contact				
Any medical contact in week before death	78	39	2.8*	1.7–4.9
Any medical contact in month before death	133	108	1.6*	1.0–2.4
Contact with GP				
Week before death	59	31	2.6*	1.5–4.7
Month before death	111	101	1.3	0.8–1.9
12 months before death	184	169	1.7	1.0–3.0
Psychiatric inpatient contact				
Week before death	13	2	6.5*	1.5–59.3
Month before death	18	4	4.5*	1.5–18.3
12 months before death	38	8	6.0*	2.5–17.4
Psychiatric outpatient contact				
Week before death	13	2	6.5*	1.5–59.3
Month before death	25	2	12.5*	3.1–109
12 months before death	59	14	6.0*	2.9–13.8
Any psychiatric contact				
Week before death	25	3	8.3*	2.5–43.1
Month before death	39	6	6.1*	2.7–18.8
12 months before death	76	20	5.0*	2.8–9.6
Medication prescribed				
On any type of medication at death	149	130	1.6*	1.0–2.6
Given prescription in month before death	104	79	1.8*	1.1–2.8
Given prescription in week before death	49	31	1.8*	1.0–3.1
On psychotropic medication at death	103	38	6.1*	3.4–11.9
Given prescription of psychotropic medication in month before death	81	28	5.1*	2.8–10.0
Given prescription of psychotropic medication in week before death	46	11	6.7*	2.8–19.2

*P < 0.05 (McNemar Test); ** 95% Confidence Interval of Odds Ratio

Question AI

What are *three* strengths and *two* weaknesses of the method of identifying the cases described in this study?

[2 marks for each strength and weakness indicated up to a maximum of 10 marks]

[Total 10 marks]

Question A2

The study described above is a case-control design. An alternative design is a cohort design. Identify and briefly explain *two* advantages and *three* disadvantages of a cohort design to investigate the factors leading to death by suicide in such a geographically defined community.

[2 marks for each answer including the explanation stated up to a maximum of 10 marks]

[Total 10 marks]

Question A3

(i)   The choice of a suitable control group is a key element in the design of a case–control study. Given the study design, involving retrospective abstraction of information from records, list *three* disadvantages of choosing the particular control group used.

[2 marks for each up to a maximum of 6 marks]

(ii)   Given the Director of Public Health's questions and using the same cases who had committed suicide, what would have been the best control group to use to answer the questions concerned?

[4 marks]

[Total 10 marks]

Question A4

(i)   The assessors who abstracted information were not blind to the coroner's conclusions (that is, the suicide verdict, or 'caseness'). Does this matter, and if so, why?

[4 marks]

(ii)   List any important risk factors not investigated by the researchers.

[6 marks]

[Total 10 marks]

Question A5

(i)   State *three* significant differences between cases and controls in the results shown in Table A1 specifically relating to life events and difficulties prior to death.

[2 marks for each up to a maximum of 6 marks]

(ii)   Give *one* factor that could have affected the accuracy of these figures and explain how this could have affected the results?

[2 marks for the reason and 2 marks for the explanation up to a maximum of 4 marks]

[Total 10 marks]

Question A6

List *five* key features from the data presented in Table A2.

[2 marks for each key feature and explanation up to a maximum of 10 marks]

[Total 10 marks]

Question A7

The Director of Public Health queried whether an intervention in the psychiatric outpatient clinic could significantly reduce the suicide rate. Assume that your local area has a similar sociodemographic and economic profile to that in the study. In view of the findings in Table A2 regarding contact with psychiatric services:

(i)   What is likely to be the overall impact of any intervention based within the psychiatric outpatient clinic on the local suicide rate?

[2 marks]

Explain briefly your reasoning, with reference to the data given.

[4 marks]

(ii)   What percentage reduction of actual suicides in those attending the outpatient psychiatric clinic within the previous month would need to be achieved to lead to a 5% reduction in suicide rate overall? Please show how you derive this.

[4 marks]

[Total 10 marks]

Question B

The figure below is extracted from a meta-analysis in a systematic review in the Cochrane Database of interventions for deliberate self-harm (the data refer to studies responding to episodes of deliberate self-harm with an intensive intervention including outreach, compared with standard clinical aftercare). The data are presented exactly as they are shown on the Cochrane Database. To be included in the meta-analysis, studies needed to be randomised trials. The results in the figure refer specifically to repetition of deliberate self-harm.

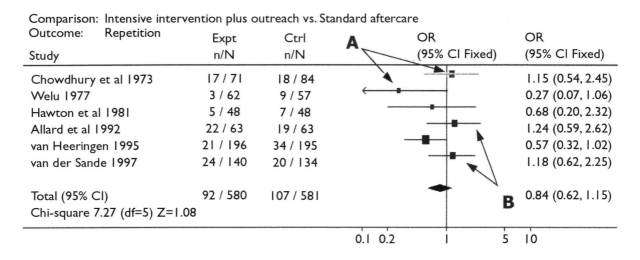

Comparison: Intensive intervention plus outreach vs. Standard aftercare					
Outcome: Repetition	Expt	Ctrl	A	OR	OR
Study	n/N	n/N		(95% CI Fixed)	(95% CI Fixed)
Chowdhury et al 1973	17 / 71	18 / 84			1.15 (0.54, 2.45)
Welu 1977	3 / 62	9 / 57			0.27 (0.07, 1.06)
Hawton et al 1981	5 / 48	7 / 48			0.68 (0.20, 2.32)
Allard et al 1992	22 / 63	19 / 63			1.24 (0.59, 2.62)
van Heeringen 1995	21 / 196	34 / 195			0.57 (0.32, 1.02)
van der Sande 1997	24 / 140	20 / 134			1.18 (0.62, 2.25)
Total (95% CI)	92 / 580	107 / 581		B	0.84 (0.62, 1.15)
Chi-square 7.27 (df=5) Z=1.08					

Figure 1.

Question BI

(i)   What is represented by the boxes marked A in Figure I?

[4 marks]

(ii)   Note that the boxes marked A in Figure I are of different sizes. What does this represent?

[2 marks]

(iii)   What is represented by the horizontal lines marked B?

[2 marks]

(iv)   How are these interpreted?

[2 marks]

[Total 10 marks]

Question B2

A meta-analysis uses data from several different studies.
One risk of doing this is excessive variability between studies in their results (that is, study heterogeneity).

(i)   What information in the figure is pertinent to the assessment of this heterogeneity?

[4 marks]

(ii)   Indicate whether the results of the studies described are homogeneous, i.e. compatible with the results of the others?

[6 marks]

[Total 10 marks]

Question B3

(i)   Point out and explain features in Figure 1, which indicate the results arising from the combination of the individual studies.

[4 marks]

(ii)   Give *three* main results of the meta-analysis, omitting the answers you have given to the questions above.

[2 marks for each answer up to a maximum of 6 marks]

[Total 10 marks]

Model answers by Anne Cahill

Question A1

Strengths

1. The study attempts to identify a complete case series of people dying by suicide, within a defined time period and defined geographical area. In general, the ascertainment of a complete case series is less subject to bias than the selection of a subset of cases.

2. The case series initially includes people recorded as having died of 'undetermined injury' as well as definite suicides. This is a strength because coroners are known to require a high degree of certainty before the verdict of suicide is given – some completed suicides will therefore receive a verdict of 'undetermined injury' and will not be included if only individuals with a coroner's verdict of suicide are examined.

3. 'Undetermined injuries' are then examined by the researchers in closer detail, eliminating those who probably did not die by suicide. The final case series consists therefore of 'suicides, and probable suicides'.

Weaknesses

1. Because coroners' verdicts are not totally accurate, some cases of suicide may have been misclassified, e.g. some deaths apparently by natural causes may have in fact been suicides but will not be included in the case series.

2. The deaths are identified from regional records. Individuals who travelled outside the region prior to suicide may therefore have been omitted from the case series.

Question A2

Advantages

1. A cohort study can be prospective – a cohort is identified at a time before the critical outcome has occurred, and followed forward in time. Data on factors thought to have predictive value as to the outcome can be collected prospectively. The process of collecting data on predictor variables may thus be less subject to bias – data can be collected with equal accuracy for both eventual cases and their controls, and the quality of the information collected will not be biased by knowledge of the outcome.

2. There are less problems in selecting an appropriate control group in a cohort study design. All individuals within the cohort in whom the outcome does not occur are compared with the individuals in whom it does. It may still be necessary to consider confounding variables – but overall this process is less subject to bias than the matching procedures adopted in case–control studies.

Disadvantages

1. Suicide is a rare outcome, so a large inception cohort would be needed to identify enough cases of suicide, to produce a study of sufficient power to make meaningful comparisons. The area has a modest sized population (471,000) and a large enough cohort would not be easily available.

2. A prospective cohort study of factors predicting suicide would by definition require a very long timescale, in order to follow each and every individual included until the time of their death. There would probably be considerable loss to follow-up due to people moving away, and it would also be very resource intensive.

3. A huge amount of information would have to be gathered about a very large number of people, the vast majority of whom would not have the outcome of interest.

Question A3

(i)

1. Only a small subset of deaths is reported to the coroner – those thought to require investigation – so the causes of death in the control group are atypical of the general population. They have presumably also died at an atypically young age, since suicide is a cause of premature death. The study comparisons are thus difficult to interpret as the control group is not typical of the population at large.

2. People who have died in an atypical way may also differ systematically from the general population in the types of ante-mortem information available in medical records. The availability of this information is crucial to this study.

3. There does not appear to be the same scrutiny of coroners' records to verify the cause of death in the selection of the control group. The study is therefore more reliant on the accuracy of coroners' verdicts in the case of the control group – it may be that some cases of suicide have been misclassified and included in this group.

(ii)
The best control group might be a group of living individuals, matched for age, sex and also for some carefully defined measure of psychiatric diagnosis/morbidity. This would allow you to compare people who died by suicide with a set of controls exhibiting the same levels of psychiatric difficulty, but who have not died by suicide.

Question A4

(i)
Yes, because knowledge of cause of death may have introduced bias into the process of abstracting the information on predictor variables, e.g. researchers may have looked more assiduously for evidence of adverse life events or other factors believed to be associated with suicide in people known to have died by suicide.

(ii)
Does the person have a serious physical illness?
Have they expressed suicidal ideas or intent in the time leading up to suicide?
Have they recently been detained under a section of the Mental Health Act?
Have they defaulted from psychiatric services?
Social class and occupation.
Also – age and sex not investigated, as included in matching procedures.

Question A5

(i)
Cases were more likely than controls to have suffered
1. recent separation
2. financial difficulties
3. relationship difficulties.

(ii)
Accuracy could have been affected by fuller documentation of life events in the cases than in the controls, e.g. controls may have been less likely to mention life events of this nature to any doctor or GP since they might not have seemed so relevant to their medical problems, or they may have been less likely to have attended a doctor at all. This would artificially inflate the apparent role of such events among cases.

Question A6

Cases, as compared with controls, were
1. more likely to have been taking psychotropic medication at time of death (nearly 50% of cases, as opposed to 18% of controls)
2. more likely to have had psychiatric out-patient contact in time before death (all 3 time intervals)
3. more likely to have had psychiatric in-patient contact in time before death (all 3 time intervals)
4. GP contact in the week before death is higher in cases than controls, but GP contact within the longer time intervals (previous month and previous year) does not distinguish cases and controls
5. 136 of the 212 people (64%) who died by suicide had no contact with any psychiatric service in the year before death.

Question A7

(i)
At the very best, a reduction in the overall suicide rate of 27.8%.
   Assuming all cases can be picked up and prevented when they attend clinic, in the 12 months before they might otherwise take their own life, this would prevent 59/212 suicides = 27.8%. Actual impact will be much less, as clearly this level of prevention not possible in practice.

(ii)

Between 42 and 43%.

The total number of suicides in the time interval is 212 and 5% of 212 = 10.6.

Number of eventual suicides who attend OPC in month before death = 25.

Then 10.6/25 = 42.4

Question B1

(i)
The boxes represent the point estimate of the difference between experimental and control groups in each study, expressed in the form of an odds ratio.

(ii)
The size of the box represents the number of subjects in each study. Bigger study = bigger box.

(iii)
These lines represent the 95% confidence interval of the odds ratio, in each study.

(iv)
There is a 95% chance that the true value of the difference between the groups lies between the two extremes represented by the 95% confidence intervals.

Question B2

(i)
Heterogeneity can be judged by looking at the degree of overlap between the confidence intervals of the different studies.

(ii)
This can be judged graphically by attempting to draw a line which intersects each of the 95% confidence intervals; if this is impossible the studies are heterogeneous. Given that such a line can be drawn, the results of the studies are homogeneous.

Question B3

(i)
The diamond shaped box at the bottom is a graphic representation of the combined results. Its value represents a pooled odds ratio of 0.84 with 95% confidence intervals 0.62–1.15. The chi square statistic quoted at the bottom also relates to the combined result, indicating the degree of deviation from a chance distribution, and giving a measure of statistical significance in the form of a Z score.

(ii)
1.   There have only been six randomised controlled trials of interventions for deliberate self-harm between 1973 and 1997, and only 199 patients are included in total.

2.   There is a small reduction in repetitions of deliberate self-harm in the intensive intervention group as compared with the control group when the results of the studies are pooled.

3.   However, the 95% confidence interval of the pooled estimate spans the value 1.00 (line of no effect), as indeed do all of the 95% confidence intervals for the individual studies. We therefore cannot conclude that the effect is not due to chance.

MRCPsych Part II Examination
Critical Review Paper
Autumn 2001

Please read the instructions carefully before going further.

Instructions

1. This examination lasts for 90 minutes.
2. The paper has TWO questions, Question A and Question B. You must attempt ALL parts of BOTH questions.
3. A total of 100 marks has been allocated to the whole paper. Each part of each question is worth 10 marks. Therefore, Question A is worth 70 marks, and Question B is worth 30 marks.
4. In answering Question A, candidates may wish to glance briefly at the questions they are asked to answer (on pages 75–78 of the paper), before reading the details of the research (described on pages 72–75).
5. Candidates are advised to bring a calculator to the examination hall for this paper. Candidates are only permitted to take a noiseless, cordless, pocket-sized non-programmable calculator WITHOUT printout or graphic/word display facilities.
6. Please do not remove this Examination paper from the Examination Room.

Question A

Scenario

Mr Y is a 29 year old man who was struck from behind while driving his car, which was stationary, while waiting to enter a roundabout. He sustained a broken leg, neck sprain and a cut forehead and was admitted to hospital because of his injuries. He was found to be highly distressed and hypervigilant, exhibiting symptoms of panic and fear of dying with signs of sympathetic overarousal. He was discharged 2 weeks following the admission. He was not seen by any mental health service personnel at any time during the admission.

You are an SHO in liaison psychiatry in an Accident & Emergency Department in which all patients with emotional problems following accidents are assessed by a psychiatrist. You had read that ventilation of feelings at the time of the accident might be of benefit in aiding recovery. You perform a literature search and find the following paper.

Mayou RA, Ehlers A and Hobbs M. Psychological debriefing for road traffic accident victims. *British Journal of Psychiatry*, 2000; **176**, 589–593.

The methods and results are summarised below.

The paper

The paper describes a follow-up study of patients who had been admitted to hospital immediately following a road traffic accident. Half the group had received a debriefing intervention following the accident, whereas the remainder had only received conventional physical treatment.

Methods

The subjects were consecutive victims of road accidents admitted to a hospital in Oxford. All those who had no memory of the accident or were intoxicated at the time of the accident were excluded. Patients were aged 16–65 years. All those who agreed to participate were allocated by a system of random numbers either to intervention or to a non-intervention control group. All allocated to the intervention group (50% of the sample subjects) were interviewed by a research worker and debriefed within 24 hours of the accident or as soon as they were physically fit to be seen. They were followed up at 4 months and again at 3 years.

Baseline measures

The following instruments were administered to all patients immediately after the interview.

Impact of Events Scale (IES), a scale that measures symptoms of intrusive perceptions and avoidance symptoms. It has been found to be significantly correlated with severity of Post-Traumatic Stress Disorder.

General Symptom Index (GSI), a semi-structured interview administered by an observer that assesses emotional distress. It covers a comprehensive array of psychiatric symptoms. High scores indicate greater morbidity.

Abbreviated Injury Severity (AIS) score – assesses both severity and site of injury.

Length of stay in hospital.

Follow-up measures

IES and GSI as above.

Problems with driving. Patients were asked whether they found road travel as a driver and as a passenger less enjoyable than before the accident. Patients assessed whether they still suffered pain from their accident on a 4-point scale. Patients rated how well they had recovered physically from their injuries on a 3-point scale.

Intervention

Subjects in the intervention group were offered a debriefing intervention, which lasted approximately I hour. This included a detailed review of the accident, the encouragement of appropriate emotional expression, and cognitive appraisal of the subjects' perceptions of the accident. The aim of the intervention was to promote the emotional and cognitive processes which, it is believed, lead to resolution of the trauma. The research workers stressed the value of talking about the experience, rather than suppressing thoughts and feelings, and the value of an early and graded return to normal travel. Subjects were given a leaflet summarising the principles of the intervention, advising consultation with the family doctor if problems persisted. GPs were informed of the study and sent a copy of this leaflet.

Statistical analyses

Scores on the IES and GSI were not normally distributed. They were log-transformed, which normalised the distributions. Changes in these scores over time were analysed with repeated measures analysis of variance (ANOVA). Differences between the intervention and control groups were tested using analysis of covariance (ANCOVA), with baseline scores as the covariates.

To investigate whether there were differential effects of the intervention, depending on the initial severity of intrusion and avoidance symptoms, patients were classified as to whether they had low (<24) or high (>25) initial IES scores. This cut-off point was chosen because it represented the top 25% of the initial IES scores. Group differences were analysed with 2-way ANCOVA, using baseline IES scores as the covariate, and intervention v. control and high v. low initial score as the between-subject factors.

Ratings for loss of enjoyment when driving or being a passenger, pain and physical problems at 3 years were analysed using t-tests. ANCOVAs were used to control for the possible effects of injury severity on the outcome measures.

Results

Of the 106 patients who had originally participated in the intervention study, 61 patients (30 from the intervention group and 31 controls) were assessed at 3 years post-intervention. Patients who responded to the 3-year follow-up did not differ from those who did not respond in terms of initial symptom severity, age, gender, marital status, social class, driver or passenger, vehicle type, length of hospital stay, history of emotional problems and initial emotional response to the accident. However, follow-up participants had been more severely injured (mean severity 1.85 v. 1.58, $t(104)=2.13$, $P=0.035$). There were no significant differences between follow-up patients who had received the debriefing intervention and controls. However, when types of injury were considered separately, it was found that the intervention group had more severe injuries of their limbs (mean severity 1.33 v 0.71, $t(59)=2.22$,

P=0.030). There was no difference between intervention (27%) and control groups (29%) in the proportion of patients classified as having high initial scores ($\chi^2(1,61)=0.42$, P=0.84).

The comparison of the scores on the questionnaires and instruments at the time of the initial assessment and the 3-year follow-up period is illustrated in Table AI.

Table AI.   Outcome of psychological debriefing v. no intervention at 3-year follow-up (The figures are means with standard deviations in brackets.)

	Intervention group		Control Group	
	Pre	3 years	Pre	3 years
Intrusion/avoidance symptoms (IES)	14.9 (13.8)	16.0 (17.6)	15.9 (11.9)	13.1 (16.7)
IES scores for patients with high initial scores (>23)	34.9 (10.3)	25.9 (13.2)	31.3 (5.7)	11.8 (17.2)
Emotional distress (GSI)	0.48 (0.54)	0.67 (0.68)	0.40 (0.31)	0.35 (0.46)
Impaired enjoyment of driving (0–3)		1.45 (1.68)		1.27 (2.07)
Impaired enjoyment of being a passenger (0–3)		1.57 (1.17)		0.75 (0.97)
Pain (0–3)		1.27 (0.98)		0.55 (0.77)
Chronic physical problems (0–2)		0.90 (0.71)		0.52 (0.57)

Intrusion and avoidance symptoms as measured by the IES were lower at the 3-year follow-up than at initial assessment (F $(1,59)=6.33$, P=0.015). The ANCOVA did not show a significant effect of intervention on IES scores at 3 years (F $(1,58)=2.03$, P=0.16). On examination of the differential effects of the intervention on patients with high and low initial IES scores the ANCOVA of IES scores at 3 years showed a significant effect of intervention (F $(1,56)=4.91$, P=0.031). There was also a significant interaction of intervention and IES group (high v. low initial scores: (F $(1,56)=4.29$, P=0.043). For those with low initial scores, there were no differences between intervention and control patients, but the intervention group had a significantly worse outcome amongst those who had high initial scores (t $(14)=2.56$. P=0.023; observed difference 0.74; 95% confidence intervals (CI) for difference 0.11–1.28).

Intervention patients with high initial IES scores had more severe injuries (2.0 v. 1.2, t $(15)=3.29$, P=0.005) and stayed marginally longer in hospital (2.2 v. 1.4, t $(15)=1.80$, P=0.092). When the injury severity for different body parts was considered separately, it emerged that the intervention group had more severe injuries of their limbs (1.6 v. 0.3, t $(15)=2.99$, P=0.009). Analyses of covariance tested whether any of these variables could account for the higher IES scores of the intervention group after 3 years. In all instances, the intervention factor remained at least marginally significant (all P<0.07).

With regard to the GSI the ANCOVA of 3-year follow-up scores, controlling for baseline scores, showed a significant effect of intervention (F $(1, 57)=5.21$, P=0.026). Patients in the intervention groups reported more severe psychiatric symptoms at follow-up (observed difference 0.08; 95% confidence intervals (CI) for difference 0.009–0.15).

With regard to other outcomes, the groups did not differ in terms of enjoyment of driving (t $(57)=0.37$, P>0.1). Those in the Intervention Group reported more severe pain (t $(59)=3.19$, P=0.002, observed difference=0.72, 95% CI for difference 0.27–1.17). The effects were the same when mean severity of injury, length of hospital stay, or injuries of limbs were controlled in analyses of covariance (all P<0.007). Patients in the Intervention Group reported having recovered less well physically than controls (t $(59)=2.33$, P=0.023, observed difference=0.38, 95% CI for difference, 0.05–0.71). In the Intervention Group, 20% described major chronic physical health problems, compared with 3.2% of the control group. The difference between the groups was only partially accounted for by differences in severity of injury, because the worse outcome for intervention subjects remained marginally significant in analyses of covariance controlling for mean injury severity, length of hospital stay or injuries to limbs (all $P < 0.07$).

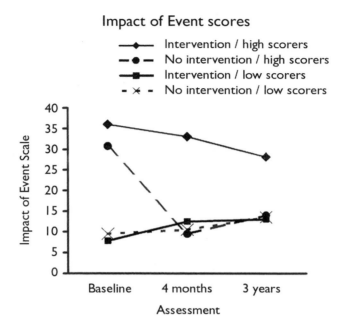

Figure A1.

Question AI

(a) What main hypothesis was tested in this paper?

[3 marks]

(b) What type of study design is this?

[4 marks]

(c) Name *two* ways in which the control group differed from the intervention group?

[3 marks for mentioning both; I mark only for mentioning one]

Question A2

(a) Give the number and percentage of patients not followed up at 3 years.

[I + I marks]

(b)   Why did the authors compare the characteristics of those who were followed up at 3 years with those who did not?

[2 marks]

(c)   From the results given by the authors how confident are you that the results indicated are valid for all the subjects?

[3 marks]

(d)   What analysis can be carried out so that one can be confident that subjects who did not respond to the 3-year follow up do not distort the results?

[2 marks]

(e)   Why is such an analysis seldom carried out?

[I mark]

Question A3

List *five* weaknesses in the study design or its implementation, given the intervention proposed. For each point you list, explain how it might affect the outcome of the study, and in which direction.

[2 marks for each up to a maximum of 10 marks]

Question A4

(a)   In the statistical analysis it is stated that the scores on the IES and the GSI questionnaires were log-transformed. Why is such a log transformation procedure carried out?

[4 marks]

(b)   If a log-transformation fails, and other transformations also fail in this regard, how else can the results be analysed?

[3 marks]

(c)   Which of the following statistical tests used in the study rely on the log-transformed IES and GSI scores to be normally distributed in order to be valid?
- *t*-tests − p values
- *t*-tests − 95% confidence intervals
- ANCOVA − p values

[I mark for each correct answer up to a maximum of 3 marks]

Question A5

(a)   In the other outcome measures it is stated that the intervention group reported different levels of pain than the standard treatment group. The figures t (59)$=$3.19, P$=$0.002, observed difference$=$0.72, 95% CI for difference, 0.27–1.17. are given. What is the null hypothesis posed for this particular comparison?

[2 marks]

(b)   Interpret the figures regarding the difference reported.

[2 marks]

(c)   What is the relative risk of harm in terms of chronic physical health if a patient receives the intervention?

[2 marks]

(d)   What is the Number Needed to Harm (NNH) of patients allocated to the intervention group? What does this figure mean?

[4 marks]

Question A6

(a)   Look at Figure A1. Give *three* main findings shown.

[2 marks for each up to a maximum of 6 marks]

(b)   Identify *two* other pieces of information which you would like to have before you would accept the conclusions as stated above?

[2 marks for each up to a maximum of 4 marks]

Question A7

(a)   Mr. Y would like to know what his chances are of having continuing psychiatric or physical symptoms 3 years after the accident. He particularly would like to know the nature of the symptoms from which he is likely to suffer. Give *two* findings from this investigation that will inform him further about these symptoms.

[2 marks for each up to a maximum of 4 marks]

(b)   He also wishes to know whether a debriefing procedure is likely to assist him in avoiding later symptoms and which ones are likely to be altered by this procedure. Give *two* findings from this investigation that will inform him about what effects would be predicted if the debriefing procedure was carried out.

For this question, assume the results in this paper are valid. Please indicate, using the figures given in Table AI, what your responses would be to these questions. No precise calculations are necessary.

[2 marks for each up to a maximum of 4 marks]

(c)   With what degree of confidence can you inform Mr. Y that the results of this investigation will have applicability in his case?

[2 marks]

Question B

You have admitted a 21-year-old woman following a third overdose within the past 6 months. A medical student in your firm has noted that her serum cholesterol concentration performed during the last admission was rather low at 4.2 mmol/l. The student has drawn your attention to a table in the following paper, and suggested that giving the patient a high cholesterol diet may be an appropriate treatment to reduce further suicidal gestures.

Garland M, Hickey D, Corvin A, Golden J, Fitzpatrick P, Cunningham S, Walsh, N. Total serum cholesterol in relation to psychological correlates in parasuicide. *British Journal of Psychiatry* 2000; **177**: 77–83

In this study, the total serum cholesterol and self-rated scores for impulsivity, depression, and suicidal intent were measured in 100 consecutive patients following parasuicide, and pair-matched with normal and psychiatric control groups.

The following table is adapted from the paper, and displays part of the results of the multiple regression analysis to determine independent factors associated with cholesterol levels within the three groups.

Table BI. Multivariate analysis to determine independent factors associated with serum cholesterol level in the three groups (N.B. results of some variables omitted)

Variable	Variable sub-category	Number	Mean cholesterol (mmol/l)	Adjusted F value
Group	DSH	100	4.41 (1.02)	28.76**
	Normal	100	4.69 (0.97)	
	Psychiatric	100	4.95 (1.07)	
Age (years)	16–26	100	4.22 (0.73)	74.22**
	27–35	101	4.76 (1.07)	
	>35	99	5.07 (1.09)	
Social class	I	11	4.89 (1.17)	—
	II	63	4.57 (0.85)	3.94*
	III	125	4.57 (1.02)	10.93**
	IV	53	5.03 (1.83)	31.96**
	V	48	4.69 (1.05)	—
Previous history of DSH	Yes	50	4.50 (1.20)	8.81**
	No	250	4.72 (0.99)	
BIS-II non-planning sub-scale 3	0–24	109	4.81 (0.99)	10.58**
	25–29	92	4.67 (1.07)	—
	>29	99	4.56 (1.07)	9.23**
BIS-II score attentional sub-scale 1	0–17	96	4.74 (1.03)	—
	18–21	104	4.61 (1.02)	
	>21	100	4.70 (1.08)	
BIS-II score Motor sub-scale 2	0–20	97	5.04 (1.16)	74.99**
	21–25	103	4.51 (0.84)	18.35**
	>25	100	4.51 (1.01)	10.58**

— = *non-significant* factors; *p < 0.05; **p < 0.01.

BIS-II – The Barrett Impulsivity Scale designed to measure impulsivity. Sub-scale 3 (non-planning impulsivity) measures the tendency to make decisions without planning, sub-scale 1 (attentional impulsivity) measures level of concentration and sub-scale 2 (motor impulsivity) measures the tendency to do things without thinking. A high score represents a high level of impulsivity in the domain concerned.

Question B1

(a)   Why was multivariate analysis needed in this study? (i.e. why was univariate analysis not sufficient?)

[2 marks]

(b)

(i)   Explain why age was included as a variable in the analysis, although the aim of the study was to examine the relationship between serum cholesterol level and psychological parameters in parasuicide?

(ii)   What do we call this type of variable (as exemplified by age in this study)?

(iii)   How does this variable affect the conclusions?

[4 marks]

(c)   In the last column of Table BI, the adjusted F value for age was 74.22 and the footnotes indicate $p < 0.01$. Explain how this enables us to draw some conclusions about the relationship between age and cholesterol levels?

[4 marks]

Question B2

List *five* important features from Table BI. (Exclude the result on age, which has already been explored in question BI.) *More marks will be given for indicating the most important findings first in your answer.*

[2 marks for each up to a maximum of 10 marks]

Question B3

Does this study show conclusively that a low cholesterol concentration causes parasuicide?

[1 mark]

(b)   Give *three* other possible explanations (other than parasuicide directly caused by low cholesterol) to explain the apparent association between deliberate self-harm and cholesterol levels?

[2 marks for each up to a maximum of 6 marks]

(c)   Would you recommend that a high cholesterol diet be used in the management of this patient based on this study?

[3 marks]

Model answers by Clementine Maddock and Matthew Hotopf

Question A1

(a)
Psychological debriefing following a road traffic accident reduces post-traumatic stress and psychological symptoms at 3 years.

(b)
Randomised controlled trial.

(c)
Intervention group had more severe injuries of their limbs.

Intervention group had higher mean emotional distress (GSI) scores at baseline.

Question A2

(a)
45/106 (42%) were lost to follow-up.

(b)
In order to explore possible bias, which may be introduced if the follow-up group differ significantly in terms of possible confounders such as age and gender. As subjects drop out of a randomised controlled trial, the treatment and control groups depart from the balanced groups created at randomisation.

(c)
Most of the factors considered did not differ between those followed up and those who didn't respond. However, follow-up participants had been more severely injured, which, if we assume severity of injury is associated with psychological symptoms, may have resulted in the mean 3-year scores being higher than they would have been if all subjects had responded to follow-up.

(d)
Intention to treat analysis. This includes all the patients who started the study in the final analysis. Drop-outs are either considered as treatment failures, or the last observation carried forward is used for the final analysis. If drop-outs are excluded, then results tend to over-estimate the effects of treatment.

(e)
Investigators are less likely to find an effect of treatment if all drop-outs are considered treatment failures.

Question A3

1. It is not stated if the randomisation list was concealed. The person enrolling the patient in the study should not be able to predict which group the patient will be randomly allocated to, as that might introduce bias, which tends to exaggerate treatment effects.

2. The groups differed at the start of the trial – the intervention group had more severe injuries, which may bias results in favour of the control group.

3. It is not clear whether the investigators were blind to the treatment group of patients at the point of assessment. The text states that the GSI is a semi-structured interview administered by an observer, and so bias may have been introduced at assessment in favour of the intervention group.

4. There is a large loss to follow-up (42%). As treatment drop-outs are excluded from the analysis, this is likely to over-estimate the effect of the intervention.

5. A stratified block randomisation procedure could have been carried out whereby patients are randomised in blocks according to a particular characteristic, e.g. injury severity, so that this is balanced across intervention and control groups. This would have reduced the bias in favour of the control group (who had less severe injuries), in this case.

Question A4

(a)
The scores on the IES and GSI were not normally distributed and so they were log-transformed, which normalised the distribution and allowed more robust parametric statistical tests to be applied, e.g. ANOVA or ANCOVA.

(b)
If a normal distribution cannot be achieved, then non-parametric tests can be used, e.g. Mann–Whitney U test, Kruskal–Wallis.

(c)
All 3 tests require a normal distribution.

Question A5

(a)
The null hypothesis is that there is no difference between the mean levels of pain reported in the control and intervention groups.

(b)
The level of pain reported by the intervention group was 0.72 points higher than the control group. This is a statistically significant result as the confidence interval does not cross 0.

(c)

$$\text{Relative risk harm} = \frac{\text{experimental event risk (EER)}}{\text{control event risk (CER)}}$$

$$= \frac{0.200}{0.032} \text{ or } \frac{2.0}{3.2}$$

$$= 6.25$$

(d)
$$\text{Number needed to harm (NNH)} = \frac{1}{\text{absolute risk increase}}$$

$$= \frac{1}{\text{EER} - \text{CER}}$$

$$= \frac{1}{0.2 - 0.032}$$

$$= 5.9$$

Therefore, 6 people would need to receive the intervention for 1 extra person to have chronic physical health problems.

Question A6

(a)
1. Patients who scored higher than 24 on the IES at baseline and received debriefing showed a slight decline in PTSD symptoms although they are still scoring highly at 3 years.

2. In contrast, patients who scored higher than 24 on the IES at baseline, who did NOT receive debriefing, show a dramatic reduction in PTSD symptoms by 4 months which is maintained at 3 years.

3. Patients who scored lower than 24 on the initial IES showed a similar low level of symptoms at 4 months and 3 years, regardless of whether or not they had received debriefing.

(b)
Statistically significant interaction term.
Evidence that the subgroup analysis was based on an *a priori* hypothesis.

Question A7

(a)

Mr Y is very unlikely to suffer from chronic major physical health problems at 3 years – he has a 3 in 100 chance of doing so.

Most PTSD symptoms improve by 4 months.

(b)

Mr Y should be advised against debriefing on the basis of this study. He is likely to maintain many of his PTSD symptoms at 3 years with debriefing, whereas they are likely to resolve to low levels without debriefing.

He is likely to experience greater emotional distress at 3 years than at present if debriefing is carried out.

(c)

Mr Y experienced quite a severe injury (broken leg) and PTSD symptoms that we assume would score highly on the IES. In this case, it would seem that the results of this paper are applicable to him. However, the validity of this paper has been questioned by the weaknesses identified in question A3. Overall, there is no evidence that debriefing confers any benefit, and it may possibly be harmful, and so he should be advised against it.

Question BI

(a)

Univariate analysis examines the relationship between the dependent variable and one possible independent variable at a time. In this case, there is more than one independent variable, and so multivariate analysis is used to examine the relationship between the dependent variable and several independent variables together.

(b)

(i)   Age is included as a variable, as lower age might feasibly be associated with both lower cholesterol levels and higher levels of deliberate self-harm (DSH).

(ii) This is a confounding variable.

(iii) A confounder is an independent variable associated with both the explanatory variable and the outcome variable.

(c)

Younger people have lower cholesterol levels and older people have higher cholesterol levels. As $p < 0.01$, this tells us that there is a less than 1 in 100 possibility that the association between age and cholesterol levels could have occurred by chance alone.

Question B2

There is a statistically significant difference between cholesterol levels in DSH, normal and psychiatric patients, with DSH patients having lower levels than the other two groups.

High levels of motor impulsivity are associated with lower cholesterol levels and this finding is statistically significant at the 1% level.

A high level of non-planning impulsivity is associated with lower cholesterol levels in patients.

Patients with a previous history of DSH have lower cholesterol levels.

Attentional impulsivity scores are not associated with cholesterol levels.

Question B3

(a)

No – this study shows an association not causation.

(b)

1.   Confounding – a factor not identified, e.g. lower saturated fat consumption is responsible for both lower cholesterol levels and higher rates of self-harm.

2. Chance – a type 1 error – a statistically significant association may have occurred by chance.

3. Reverse causality – DSH results in lower cholesterol levels, e.g. paracetamol affects cholesterol levels.

(c)
No. There is no evidence of causation, and the differences in cholesterol levels identified may be statistically significant, but they are not clinically significant. In addition, a high cholesterol diet is potentially harmful as it increases risk of cardiovascular disease.

MRCPsych Part II Examination
Critical Review Paper
Spring 2002

Please read the instructions carefully before going further.

Instructions

1. This examination lasts for 90 minutes.
2. The paper has TWO questions, Question A and Question B. You must attempt ALL parts of BOTH questions.
3. A total of 100 marks has been allocated to the whole paper. Each part of each question is worth 10 marks. Therefore, Question A is worth 70 marks, and Question B is worth 30 marks.
4. In answering Question A, candidates may wish to glance briefly at the questions they are asked to answer (on pages 88–90 of the paper), before reading the details of the research (described on pages 86–88).
5. Candidates are advised to bring a calculator to the examination hall for this paper. Candidates are only permitted to take a noiseless, cordless, pocket-sized non-programmable calculator WITHOUT printout or graphic/word display facilities.
6. Please do not remove this Examination paper from the Examination Room.

Question A

Prevention of recurrent depression with cognitive behaviour therapy

Fava, G.A., Rafanelli, C., Grandi, S., Conti, S. and Belluardo, P. 1998. *Archives of General Psychiatry* **55**, 816–820.

Scenario

Ms. Z, a woman aged 30, presented to the psychiatric clinic with her fourth episode of depressive illness since the age of 20. Her last episode was 2 years ago. She responded to antidepressants but after being on this treatment for four months, now wishes to stop drugs. She believes that cognitive therapy may be an effective treatment for her as she has located details of the study below following an Internet search.

The paper

The following is an extract from a paper published in 1998. The object was *"to apply this therapeutic approach (cognitive behaviour therapy (CBT)) to a sample of depressed patients, all of whom had suffered from repeated bouts of depression. The aim of the study was to compare this approach with that of standard clinical management (CM)."*

Patients

Forty-five consecutive out-patients satisfying the criteria described below who had been referred and treated in the Affective Disorders Programme of the University Bologna School of Medicine, Bologna, Italy, were enrolled in the study. The diagnosis of each patient was established by the consensus of a psychiatrist (G.A.F.) and a clinical psychologist (C.R.) independently using the Schedule for Affective Disorders and Schizophrenia. Patients had to meet the following criteria:

(1)   a current diagnosis of major depressive disorder according to the Research Diagnostic Criteria for a Selected Group of Functional disorders

(2)   3 or more episodes of depression with the immediately preceding episode being no more than $2\frac{1}{2}$ years before the onset of the present episode

(3)   a minimum 10-week remission according to the Research Diagnostic Criteria (with less than 2 symptoms present to no more than a mild degree with absence of functional impairment) between the index episode and the immediately preceding episode

(4)   a minimum global severity score of 7 for the current episode of depression

(5)   no history of manic, hypomanic or cyclothymic features

(6)   no history of active drug or alcohol abuse or dependence or of personality disorder according to DSM-IV criteria

(7)   no history of antecedent dysthymia

(8)   no active medical illness and

(9)   successful response to antidepressant drugs administered by two psychiatrists (S.G. and S.C.) according to a standardised protocol.

The latter protocol involved the use of tricyclic antidepressant drugs with gradual increase in dosage. Patients who could not tolerate tricyclic antidepressants were switched to a selective serotonin reuptake inhibitor.

After drug treatment, all patients were assessed by the same psychologist (C.R.) who had evaluated each patient on intake but who did not take part in treatment. Only patients rated as "better" or "much better" according to a global scale of improvement and who were in full remission were included in the study. Patients also had to show no sign of depressed mood after treatment according to a modified version of the Paykel Clinical Interview for Depression (CID).

All patients were treated for 3 to 5 months with full doses of antidepressant drugs after which the clinical psychologist administered the modified version of the CID. This interview covered 19 symptom areas. Each item is rated on a 1 to 7-point scale. It has been fully and independently validated for Italian populations.

Treatment

After assessment with CID, the 45 patients were randomly assigned to 1 of 2 treatment groups:

(1)   Pharmacotherapy and CBT

(2)   Pharmacotherapy and CM.

In both groups treatment consisted of ten 30-minute sessions once every other week. Antidepressant drug use was tapered at the rate of 25 mg of amitriptyline hydrochloride or its equivalent every other week and then the drugs were withdrawn completely (in the last two sessions, all patients were drug free). Discontinuation of antidepressant drug use was not feasible for 5 patients (3 in the CBT group and 2 in the CM group), and they were excluded from the study at that point. The same psychiatrist performed all the treatments in both groups.

Cognitive behavioural treatment consisted of the following 3 main ingredients:

(1)   Cognitive behavioural therapy of residual symptoms of major depression. Cognitive therapy was conducted as described by Beck et al. The psychiatrist, an experienced therapist, used strategies and techniques designed to help depressed patients correct their distorted views and maladaptive beliefs. Whenever appropriate, as in the case of residual symptoms related to anxiety, exposure strategies were planned with the patient.

(2)   Lifestyle modification. Patients were instructed that depression is merely the consequence of a maladaptive lifestyle, which does not take life stress, interpersonal friction, excessive work and inadequate rest into proper account.

(3)   Well-being therapy. In the last 2 or 3 sessions, a psychotherapeutic strategy for enhancing well-being was used. The technique is aimed at changing beliefs and attitudes detrimental to well-being, stimulating awareness of personal growth and recovery from affective illness and reinforcing behaviour promoting well-being.

Clinical management consisted of monitoring, medication tapering, reviewing the patients' clinical status and providing the patient with support and advice if necessary. In CM specific interventions such as exposure strategies, diary work and cognitive restructuring were not included.

The same clinical psychologist who had performed the previous evaluation and who was unaware of treatment assignment reassessed the 40 patients with the CID after treatment and while drug free. The patients were assessed at 3, 6, 9, 12, 15, 18, 21, and 24 months after treatment. Relapse was defined as the occurrence of a Research Diagnostic Criteria-defined episode of major depression.

Results

Forty patients (20 in each group) completed the 20-week experiment. There were no significant differences between the groups on any of the variables listed. During the two-year follow-up 5 patients

(25%) in the CBT group relapsed and 16 patients (80%) in the CM group relapsed. Of the 6 variables selected for multivariable analysis, only treatment assignment attained statistical significance.

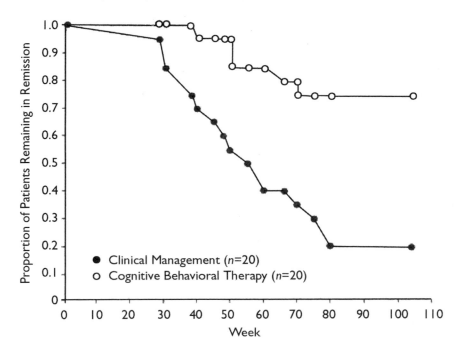

Figure 1. Proportions of depressed patients remaining in remission 2 years after cognitive behavioural therapy or clinical management.

Question A1

(a)   What is the term used for this type of study design?

[2 marks]

(b)   What precise hypothesis are the authors proposing in this study?

[3 marks]

(c)   List 5 questions you would ask to determine if this trial was carried out according to recognised ethical standards?

[1 mark for each up to a maximum of 5 marks]

Question A2

(a)   Give *five* important strengths and *five* important weaknesses of the study design. Please confine your answers to the design, not the execution of the study.

[1 mark for each up to a maximum of 10 marks]

Question A3

(a) The same therapist delivered both the cognitive therapy and the standard clinical management. Name *two* advantages and *two* disadvantages to this.

[1 mark for each up to a maximum of 4 marks]

(b) How might the study design be altered to overcome the disadvantages you have mentioned? Please list *two* methods.

[3 marks for each up to a maximum of 6 marks]

Question A4

(a) What is the term used for the graph in figure 1?

[2 marks]

(b) Give *three* main findings from the curve.

[2 marks for each up to a maximum of 6 marks]

(c) From the data described in the text, calculate the Number Needed to Treat (NNT) to prevent relapse over the next two years and explain what it means. What is the clinical significance of this result?

[2 marks]

Question A5

(a) The authors state that of the 6 variables assessed for effects on outcome only treatment allocation, presented in figure 1, attained statistical significance. Give *four* clinical variables, as distinct from social factors, related to the illness course and/or treatment, which might have been selected for analysis?

[1 mark for each up to a maximum of 4 marks]

(b) Name two of the clinical variables that you have listed (other than demographic) which are likely to have the most impact if unequally distributed between the two treatment groups, and which are likely to occur frequently.

[2 marks for each up to a maximum of 4 marks]

Indicate in what way the results of the study would be difficult to interpret if there was such unequal distribution.

[1 mark each for influence on results up to a maximum of 2 marks]

Question A6

(a)   The outcome of those patients allocated to the CBT arm is markedly better than those patients who received the CM treatment. Give 3 plausible reasons with reference to the design of the study or its execution why this should be the case. Assume that the procedures carried out in the text have been carried out as described.

[2 marks for each up to a maximum of 6 marks]

(b)   The authors stated that they excluded from analysis 5 patients who were unable to discontinue antidepressants following treatment. What effect might this have on the results?

[4 marks]

Question A7

(a)   Are the results of this study applicable to Ms Z? Please explain your reasoning.

[2 marks]

(b)   What advice would you give to Ms Z in the light of this study? In particular what would you recommend with regard to her antidepressants?

[2 marks]

(c)   Ms Z wishes to know what would be the best treatment for her to reduce the risk of relapse of depression in the years to come. What treatments would you suggest from your knowledge of this area, given the information given in this investigation?

[2 marks]

(d)   In view of the results of this paper, would you recommend that all of your patients receiving antidepressants have these withdrawn and CBT, as described in this paper, administered if they wish this, the treatment is available and cost is no object? Give *two* reasons to explain your answer.

[2 marks for each up to a maximum of 4 marks]

Question B

Nandy S., Chalmers-Watson, C., Gantley, M., Underwood, M. Referral for minor mental illness: a qualitative study. *British Journal of General Practice* 2001; **51**: 461–465.

The above paper is a qualitative study involving semi-structured interviews with general practitioners. General practitioners were sampled purposively from Health Authority lists and databases of GPs according to age, sex, country of undergraduate training, employment status, area of practice and interest in mental health. 23 out of 34 general practitioners approached agreed to be interviewed. The interviews were conducted by two GPs and involved asking open-ended questions about the responders' management of mild depression and/or anxiety. The interviews were audiotape-recorded and transcribed. A grounded theory approach was used to analyse the data by generating explanatory concepts and categories. The analytic framework was by a multi-disciplinary team. An iterative approach was adopted for data collection and analysis. It was felt that data saturation was achieved by the twenty-third interview. The results were presented to a group of 12 general practitioners just before completion of the analysis and no dissonance with their practice was felt.

Two main categories were found. They are very briefly summarised as follows.

1. Category 1: 'conduits' and 'containers' referral strategy

"Containment" strategy was adopted by GPs who tended to see minor mental illness as part of the remit of general practice and their role partly to prevent what they regarded as an inappropriate burden on other agencies.

> I've managed quite a lot myself...Most people don't want to be referred...people still want that personal contact with their GP"

"Conduit" strategy was adopted by GPs who saw themselves more in a diagnostic, and then triage role and felt that these patients are best managed by others.

> "I'm sure that the GP's job is access. The NHS is set up so it's difficult for people to get to secondary care...My job is definitely to facilitate access to appropriate services for patients."

2. Category 2: 'referrals to' and 'referrals away'

"Referrals to" were often for very specific situations (e.g. drug or alcohol addiction) or when a GP thought that a particular patient would benefit more than average from referral.

> "Many people need this [referral to a psychiatrist]. Somehow that process is needed. . . . the patient sometimes needs that even though you know that nothing particular different will happen."

"Referrals away" were often triggered by certain emotions on the doctor's part. Feelings of frustration, anger, and irritation were viewed as warning signs that the GP needed help, rather than an active decision that referral would be good for the patient.

> "a bit of bloody relief." [in reply to: 'What do you expect from referral?']

Question BI

(a)   Give one possible reason why the authors chose qualitative rather than quantitative methods in this study.

[2 marks]

(b)
(i)   Explain *in your own words* how the general practitioners were sampled in this study.

[2 marks]

(ii)   Why was random sampling not used in this study?

[2 marks]

(iii)   Give one disadvantage for this type of sampling over random sampling.

[2 marks]

(c)   What was the "response rate" of this study?

[I mark]

Comment briefly on whether it was satisfactory

[I mark]

Question B2

(a)   Briefly give I precaution the authors took to ensure the data collected were valid.

[2 marks]

(b)   Briefly give I precaution the authors took to minimise bias in data analysis

[2 marks]

(c)   Briefly give I precaution the authors took to ensure that the results obtained were credible.

[2 marks]

(d)   Did the authors begin data analysis only after all the data were collected?

[I mark]

Briefly comment on the authors' choice.

[1 mark]

(e)   Explain *in your own words* how the authors ensured that sufficient GPs had been interviewed to yield valid results.

[2 marks]

Question B3

(a)   Explain *very briefly* how the authors arrived at the two categories.

[4 marks]

(b)   Give *one* purpose for the quotations.

[2 marks]

(c)   *Very briefly* explain how this study might help you to design referral guidelines for depression from primary to secondary care.

[2 marks]

How valuable do you think these would be in practice?

[2 marks]

Model answers by Philip Shaw

Question A1

(a)
Randomised controlled trial.

(b)
The hypothesis states that there is a significantly decreased risk of relapse in depression between two groups of patients, one group receiving CBT and the other receiving standard clinical care over a 2-year period following the intervention. All subjects have a history of recurrent depressive disorder and enter the trial following successful pharmacological treatment of an acute depressive episode, at which stage medication is gradually withdrawn.

(c)
1.   Were subjects given an information sheet describing the nature and purpose of the study and any risk of the intervention (particularly the withdrawal of antidepressants)?

2.   Were subjects given adequate time to consider their decision whether or not to participate?

3.   Were subjects aware that a decision not to participate would not adversely affect their usual treatment?

4.   Were subjects informed that they could withdraw their consent at any time without any explanation?

5.   Were subjects given contact details for a member of the research team to notify in the event of an emergency relating to the trial (and an appropriate response team available for such events)?

Question A2

(a)
Strengths:
1.   The study is randomised, so participants in both wings are likely to be similar in terms of known and unknown possible confounders.

2.   The study included a clear protocol for the withdrawal of antidepressants to ensure that subjects in both groups received similar levels of decreasing medication throughout the trial.

3.   The study used well validated diagnostic and outcome measures.

4.   The proposed follow-up was both frequent and prolonged.

5.   The control group differed only in the presence of absence of the intervention (CBT package).

Weaknesses:
1.   The method of randomisation used is not clear.

2.   The CBT package includes many components which are novel, possibly specific to the individual therapist and not in standard practice. No references are given to explain the details of these interventions.

3.   There is no treatment wing that includes the long-term continuation of antidepressant medication, which in clinical practice would be the most likely treatment option.

4.   The inclusion criteria would exclude many patients seen in everyday practice, which limits the generalisability of the findings.

5.   There is no mention whether any attempt was made to blind the patients as to the hypothesis of the study. If patients were aware they were in the 'new treatment' wing this may in part account for better outcome.

Question A3

(a)
Advantages:
1.   As the same therapist delivered both treatments this partially removes the possibility that non-specific variables relating to the therapist (such as experience) could account for group differences.

2. It may also ensure that the two groups received a truly diverse treatment, with the therapist making a conscious effort not to introduce elements of one treatment modality into the other.

Disadvantages:

1. There is the possibility of bias, as the therapist designed the study and may prefer one treatment condition (the CBT wing) over the other and thus consciously or unconsciously try 'harder' with the group receiving that treatment.

2. The generalisability of the findings are limited, as they may reflect factors relating to the unique characteristics and therapeutic style of just one clinician.

(b)

1. The therapy sessions could be taped and adherence to the treatment conditions/time limits etc. checked by an independent researcher.

2. Two or more therapists could be randomly allocated to deliver each treatment condition.

Question A4

(a)
Survival curve

(b)

1. After two years 80% of patients in the CBT group and 25% of patients in the CM group did not relapse into a depressive illness.

2. The rate of relapse in the CBT group was much less than that in the CM group.

3. In the CBT group the risk of relapse was relatively constant between 30 and 80 weeks.

(c)

$NNT = 1/(\text{control event rate of } 0.80 - \text{experimental event rate of } 0.25) = 1.8$. This means that one depressive relapse in a patient over 2 years will be prevented for every 1.8 patients who receive CBT rather than standard CM. This is clearly a highly efficacious intervention in this tertiary level setting, but whether it would be as clinically effective in non-ideal settings is not clear.

Question A5

(a)

1. The type and dose of antidepressant taken at the time of the start of the trial.

2. The number of previous depressive episodes.

3. The presence of a comorbid anxiety disorder.

4. Treatment with other psychotropics such as benzodiazepines.

(b)

1. The number of previous depressive episodes may differ significantly between groups and could represent an independent underlying vulnerability to future depressive relapses.

2. If significantly more members of one group received more benzodiazepines than the other this could alter outcomes either by the drugs' positive therapeutic effects (e.g. treating some of the residual symptoms of depression) or their negative effects (e.g. decreasing the ability to perform cognitive 'homework').

Question A6

(a)

1. The cognitive component of treatment may have succeeded in changing certain styles of thought which are thought to render people vulnerable to depression – 'If I make a mistake it means I am a worthless person'.

2. The behavioural components in the lifestyle modification portion may have increased the amount of pleasurable activities subjects undertook over the follow-up period and promoted general physical health, both of which may have prevented depressive relapses.

3. The CBT package also included specific treatment for anxiety symptoms, which could contribute to decreasing future vulnerability to depressive relapses.

(b)

The failure to conduct an intention-to-treat analysis introduces possible confounds as drop-outs from each condition may not be random. If all drop-outs are considered as treatment failures this leads to a more marked increase in the relapse rate among the CBT group (from 25% to about 35%) with a less marked increase in the relapse rate in the CM group (from 80% to roughly 82%). Thus, consideration of all subjects entered into the trial leads to decrease in the strikingly different outcomes between the groups.

Question A7

(a)

Although Ms Z meets the inclusion criteria for the study there is no information on whether she also meets some of the exclusion criteria. If she had, for example, comorbid drug dependence the results of the trial are not wholly applicable to her.

(b)

I would advise her that on the basis of this study we would tentatively predict that if she stopped her antidepressants gradually and received psychiatric outpatient follow-up (which does not include the cognitive–behavioural components mentioned) she has an 80% risk of another depressive episode over a period of 2 years. If she stops her antidepressants and receives a 'cognitive–behavioural' treatment this will decrease her chances of relapse substantially, to about 25% over a 2 year period. There is no information from this trial which can inform her about the relapse rates of continuing on antidepressants in the longer term, either with standard psychiatric follow-up or in combination with CBT.

(c)

There is clear evidence on the benefits of remaining on antidepressants in the longer term in the secondary prevention of depression. This trial certainly suggests that a psychological therapy may also be a useful tool, particularly if the patient is unwilling or unable to take antidepressants. However, the trial included only small numbers of patients and was based in a rather unique setting (tertiary care) with a presumably very experienced therapist, and clearly needs replication. The weight of evidence favours her remaining on antidepressants, possibly in combination with CBT.

(d)

No. Firstly, there is no information from this study on the outcome of patients who remain on antidepressants for a longer period of time either with just standard psychiatric follow-up or in combination with CBT.

Secondly, a large proportion, if not most of the depressed patients, in my CMHT would not meet the inclusion criteria (most have not had at least three previous episodes of depression and few are in remission) but would meet the exclusion criteria (especially drug and alcohol misuse/personality disorder/medical conditions). Thus, the findings of this study do not apply to them.

Question B1

(a)

A qualitative approach is used as the study attempts to provide an understanding of the rather open-ended research question on the nature of the beliefs and attitudes that underlie the referral behaviour of GPs.

(b)

(i) GPs were sampled in a non-random manner, with GPs chosen on the basis of certain characteristics (such as gender, training).

(ii) Random sampling was not used as the authors wanted to ensure that their sample included a diverse range of GPs who varied on these potentially theoretically important characteristics. If a random sampling strategy was used the sample could, through the play of chance, include, for example, only male GPs.

(iii) As the sample of GPs were chosen on the basis of the characteristics which the researchers believe are of potential theoretical importance, the results may not be generalisable beyond that sample. A random sample would not be selected on the basis of such a priori assumptions or beliefs and may reflect more accurately the 'average' practice of GPs.

(c)

The response rate was roughly 67%.

It is unclear whether this is satisfactory as the authors do not give any data on the characteristics of the GPs who declined to participate. For example, many GPs who are not interested in mental health may have refused, thus frustrating the attempts to include this group in the sample.

Question B2

(a)
The interviewers asked open-ended questions, which allowed the GPs to answer freely on their attitudes, beliefs and referral behaviour, rather than using a closed question style of interview/questionnaire which would be based on the researchers' beliefs about referral attitudes and behaviour.

(b)
To avoid bias the team of researchers developing the explanatory categories included members of other professions allied to medicine and not just the two GPs who had collected the data.

(c)
The preliminary results were presented to a smaller group of GPs to ensure that the interpretation of the initial interviews was consistent with their own experience.

(d)
No.
   The use of the iterative method of data analysis means that the nature of the analysis, particularly the explanatory concepts which are generated, can be influenced and guided by information and results obtained as the study progresses.

(e)
Data collection was stopped once the new information did not yield any new explanatory concepts or knowledge about the inter-relationships between these concepts. The results at this stage were presented to a smaller group of GPs, in part presumably to ensure that there were no major omissions in the concepts already generated to explain referral behaviour.

Question B3

(a)
Through a constant comparison of one interview with another, certain themes emerged along with links between these themes. The two categories will have emerged frequently, acting as core categories to which the other subcategories will have been linked.

(b)
The quotes are examples of the raw data and illustrate the abstracted explanatory concepts, making them more credible.

(c)
Relevant guidelines should be based on a valid model of current attitudes to referral to secondary care, and build upon the knowledge and attitudes that already exist among GPs.
   Such guidelines are potentially very important, given that referrals from GPs are the major route of entry to secondary care. Guidelines building on existing practice and attitudes may be more likely to succeed.

MRCPsych Part II Examination
Critical Review Paper
Autumn 2002

Please read the instructions carefully before going further.

Instructions

1. This examination lasts for 90 minutes.
2. The paper has TWO questions, Question A and Question B, *each of which should be answered using separate answer booklets as indicated.*
3. You must *attempt* ALL parts of BOTH questions.
4. A total of 100 marks has been allocated to the whole paper. Each part of each question is worth 10 marks. Therefore, Question A is worth 70 marks, and Question B is worth 30 marks.
5. In answering Question A, candidates may wish to glance briefly at the questions they are asked to answer (on pages 103–106 of the paper), before reading the details of the research (described on pages 100–103).
6. Where you give more than the requested number of answers, you will only be marked on that number, e.g. If you are asked for 5 examples and give 6, you will only be marked on the first 5.
7. Candidates are advised to bring a calculator to the examination hall for this paper. Candidates are only permitted to take a noiseless, cordless, pocket-sized non-programmable calculator WITHOUT printout or graphic/word display facilities.
6. Please do not remove this Examination paper from the Examination Room.

Question A

Counselling

Scenario

As a consultant psychiatrist, you discuss issues around counselling and cognitive behaviour therapy at a local postgraduate meeting with local general practitioners. Amongst them is Dr Smith, a single-handed general practitioner with a list size of about 2,000 patients in a rural area in Scotland. He finds that he is spending much time providing care to patients with depression, and is enthusiastic to set up either non-directive counselling or cognitive behaviour therapy for such patients in his surgery. He draws your attention to the following papers on the economic analysis of such services in the British Medical Journal and asks you whether they indicate that setting up such services in his practice would save him money. (N.B. The two papers were published together and reported on the findings from the same study.)

1. Ward, E., King, M., Lloyd, M., Bower, P., Sibbald, B., Farrelly, S., *et al* (2000) Randomised controlled trial of non-directive counselling, cognitive-behaviour therapy, and usual general practitioner care for patients with depression. I. *BMJ* **321**: 1383–8.

2. Bower, P., Byford, S., Sibbald, B., Ward, E., King, M., Lloyd, M., *et al* (2000) Randomised controlled trial of non-directive counselling, cognitive-behaviour therapy and usual general practitioner care for patients with depression. II. BMJ **321**: 1389–92.

The methods and results of the papers are summarised below, with selective emphasis on aspects of economic analysis.

Paper

Methods

Patient recruitment and randomisation

Patients were recruited from February 1996 to November 1997 from 13 general practices in north London and 11 practices in greater Manchester. General practitioners were asked to refer all patients suffering from depression or mixed depression and anxiety for whom they believed a brief psychological intervention was necessary. Inclusion criteria were aged 18 years or over, and a Beck depression inventory score of $\geqslant 14$. All patients currently taking antidepressants were excluded. There were other exclusion criteria which are omitted here.

After the assessment, the researcher took each patient through the explanations about treatments and the allocation procedure. Participants were encouraged to accept randomisation to 3 groups (3-way group): usual general practitioner care, cognitive behaviour therapy and non-directive therapy. Those who continued to express a strong preference were allowed to choose their treatment (preference group). Randomisation used numbered sealed, opaque envelopes and was blocked and stratified on severity (high (>23) or low (14–22) on the Beck depression inventory).

About 9 months into the trial, the preference arms for counselling and cognitive-behaviour therapy were close to being filled. The research decided to offer new patients with a preference for psychological therapy the choice of randomisation between the two therapies (2-way group). The results of this 2-way group will not be further considered in this summary.

Sample size calculation

Sixty-five (65) patients in each group were needed to detect a mean difference in outcome between the groups of 3.5 in Beck depression inventory score (estimated SD = 8) at 90% power and a 5% level of significance.

Interventions

Six counsellors and three psychologists took part in London, as did eight counsellors and nine psychologists in Manchester. All counsellors had the necessary qualifications and experience to be accredited by the British Association for Counselling, and follow a manual on non-directive approach based on the work of Rogers. All cognitive-behaviour therapists were psychologists who had the necessary qualifications and experience for accreditation by the British Association for Behavioural and Cognitive Psychotherapists, and complied with a problem formulation and staged intervention approach. The therapists agreed to one hour of supervision for every six hours of patient contact time. Patients were offered six sessions initially, with a maximum of 12. Appointments were usually provided on a weekly basis at the surgery lasting about 50 minutes each. Participants allocated to psychological therapy were free to see their general practitioner as usual, but the doctors were requested to refrain from routinely prescribing antidepressants for these patients.

Patients allocated to the control group were treated by general practitioners according to their usual practice, but were asked to refrain from referral for psychological interventions unless this was imperative.

Outcome measures

1. Clinical

The primary clinical outcome measure is the Beck depression inventory (a self-reported inventory). Participants who refused face-to-face contact were allowed postal follow-up. Participants were assessed at referral, 4 months and 12 months. Assessors were not blind to the allocated treatment.

2. Direct cost

Two psychologists and a general practitioner collected data from general practice medical records for the 12 months before and after referral to the study on general practitioner and practice nurse consultations, hospital referrals and use of psychotropic drugs and private health services. Data were also collected from patients' self-reports at baseline, 4 months and 12 months, on visits to health professionals, hospital referrals and use of prescribed drugs. For direct non-treatment costs, only 4 patients reported child care costs, and few patients reported travel costs to secondary care. Hence, they are ignored and only the travel costs to primary care professionals and to the psychological therapy sessions were included.

3. Indirect costs

The cost of production losses was calculated from information gathered by face to face or postal interviews. Data included employment status, weeks worked, current wage rate, and an estimate of time lost from work through illness.

Unit costs were determined for the financial year 1997–8 from a variety of sources (e.g. British National Formulary, databases of Personal Social Services Research Unit). Generic drug prices were used. Travel costs were based either on self-reported fares or mileage (with unit cost supplied by the Automobile Association). The cost of time off work was based on self-reported annual, monthly, or weekly pay before tax.

Discounting was considered unnecessary in this study.

Results

Patient sample

Six hundred and twenty seven (627) patients were referred by general practices. 464 fulfilled the study criteria for inclusion. 197 patients were randomised in the 3-way group, 137 patients in the preference group, and 130 patients in the 2-way group.

Only the results in the 3-way group will be summarised. Tables 1–2 summarise the results on the clinical outcome and costs respectively. Table 3 gives the result on univariate sensitivity analysis on the total costs for the following scenarios: if full costs of missed appointments in primary care and specialist facilities were included; if the most expensive alternative drugs were used; use of national reported average wage rather than self reported wages.

Table 1. Outcomes of Beck depression inventory scores

Time	Beck depression inventory [mean (SD) scores] (N.B. Last observation carried forward data)					
	Cognitive-behavioural therapy ($n=63$)		Non-directive counselling ($n=67$)		Usual GP care ($n=67$)	
	No.	Mean (SD)	No.	Mean (SD)	No.	Mean (SD)
Baseline	63	27.6 (8.4)	67	25.4 (8.6)	67	26.5 (8.9)
4 months	56	14.3 (10.8)	62	12.9 (9.3)	62	18.3 (12.4)
12 months	50	11.4 (10.8)	58	11.8 (9.6)	57	12.1 (10.3)

Overall time by group interaction: Wilks $\lambda=0.923$; F$=3.874$; df$=4$, 380; p$=0.004$.
Differences in scores of time by group (baseline to 12 months): F$=1.41$; df$=2$, 191; p$=0.25$.
Differences in scores of time by group (baseline to 4 months): F$=4.91$; df$=2$, 191; p$=0.008$.
Differences in scores of time by group (4 months to 12 months): F$=5.29$; df$=2$, 191; p$=0.006$.

Table 2. Costs (£) for usual general practitioner care and two psychological therapies for depression at 4 and 12 months follow-up

	Usual GP care	Cognitive behaviour therapy		Non-directive counselling	
	Mean (SD)	Mean (SD)	Mean (95% CI) difference from GP care	Mean (SD)	Mean (95% CI) difference from GP care
Cost at 4 months					
Direct costs	244.0 (597.5)	215.5 (108.6)	28.5 (−119.6 to 176.6)	257.5 (356.7)	−13.5 (−181.7 to 154.7)
Indirect costs	383.7 (1194.3)	286.1 (701.3)	97.6 (−245.1 to 440.25)	444.4 (1127.2)	−60.7 (−457.6 to 336.1)
Total costs	627.7 (1359.8)	501.6 (715.3)	126.1 (−254.5 to 506.7)	701.9 (1228.4)	−74.2 (−517.1 to 368.6)
Cost at 12 months					
Direct costs	472.9 (779.3)	448.9 (471.6)	24.0 (−201.3 to 249.3)	501.4 (614.8)	−28.5 (−268.4 to 211.3)
Indirect costs	744.7 (1796.4)	611.6 (1370.4)	133.1 (−424.0 to 690.2)	897.2 (2336.1)	−152.5 (−864.7 to 559.6)
Total costs	1217.5 (2013.0)	1060.5 (1471.1)	157 (−458.0 to 772.2)	1398.6 (2474.1)	−181.1 (−951.9 to 598.7)

Table 3. Sensitivity analysis for one year total costs for usual general practitioner care and two psychological therapies for depression

	Mean (SD) costs (£)			
	Usual GP care (n=67)	Cognitive behaviour therapy (n=63)	Non-directive counselling (n=67)	Analysis of variance
Main analysis	1217.5 (2013.0)	1060.5 (1471.1)	1398.6 (2474.1)	p=0.63
Non-attendance included	1227.4 (2014.3)	1072.4 (1471.9)	1415.1 (2475.9)	p=0.63
Most expensive alternative drug	1218.7 (2015.0)	1060.7 (1471.2)	1398.8 (2474.1)	p=0.64
National wage rate	2526.5 (3042.0)	2034.8 (2629.3)	2750.9 (4155.3)	p=0.46

Question A1

Regarding randomisation *in this study*, briefly:

(a) explain the main purpose of randomisation.

[2 marks]

(b) give one advantage of preference randomisation compared to the standard randomisation procedure.

[2 marks]

(c)   explain why block randomisation was used,

[2 marks]

and comment whether block randomisation has achieved its purpose in this study.

[1 mark]

(d)   explain why stratified randomisation was used,

[1 mark]

and explain why the authors used Beck depression inventory as the criterion for stratification.

[2 marks]

Question A2

Regarding sample size calculation *in this study*

(a)   Would the number of subjects required be increased, decreased or unchanged if

(i)   the mean difference in outcome Beck depression inventory score between the groups that they expected to detect, was increased to 7;
(ii)   the level of significance required is 1%;
(iii)   the power required was 80%?

[1 mark for each up to a maximum of 3 marks] *(N.B. No calculations necessary)*

(b)   Dr Smith did not understand what "power" means. Explain this term to him simply in the context of this study.

[4 marks]

(c)   Look at the data from Tables 1 and 2 and briefly comment on the variability of Beck depression inventory scores compared to the data on costs.

[3 marks]

Question A3

(a)   Summarise the main results from Beck depression inventory scores in Table 1.

[2 marks for each result up to a maximum of 6 marks]

(b)   From the statistical results given in the footnote of Table I, can we conclude definitely that the cognitive-behavioural therapy group improved significantly more than the usual GP care group between baseline and 4 months?

[2 marks]

Explain your answer.

[2 marks]

Question A4

(a)   Which one of the following 4 types of economic analyses best describes this study overall: cost-benefit analysis, cost-effectiveness analysis, cost-utility analysis, and cost-minimisation analysis?

[2 marks]

(b)   Briefly explain your choice.

[2 marks]

(c)   Briefly state why this study does not fall into each of the other 3 types of economic analyses.

[2 marks each up to a maximum of 6 marks]

Question A5

Read the direct and indirect costs subsections under the "outcome measures" section.

(a)   The authors considered discounting but decided it was not necessary. Briefly explain what discounting is,

[I mark]

and why it was not necessary in this study.

[2 marks]

(b)   Comment on the way the authors estimated production losses.

[3 marks]

(c)   Examine Table 2 carefully.
Briefly summarise the results comparing the three types of care
(i)   at 4 months.

[2 marks]

(ii)   at 12 months.

[2 marks]

Question A6

Examine Table 3.

(a)   What is the purpose of sensitivity analysis in this study?

[2 marks]

(b)   Briefly summarise the results in Table 3, commenting on the meaning of the p value in the last column.

[1 mark for each up to a maximum of 3 marks]

(c)
(i)   What is the main disadvantage of *univariate* sensitivity analysis?

[1 mark]

(ii)   Indicate how this affects your interpretation of Table 3.

[2 marks]

(d)   If the cost of therapists' salaries were to be increased, in which direction would it affect the results?

[2 marks]

Question A7

Consider Dr Smith's original question.

(a)   Succinctly summarise the *main* conclusion of this paper in non-technical terms (preferably in no more than 40 words).

[3 marks]

(b)   Can the study findings be applied to Dr Smith's practice?

[1 mark]

Give 3 reasons for your answer.

[2 marks each up to a maximum of 6 marks]

Question B

Mortality

Pulska, T., Pahkala, K., Laippala, P., Kivela, S.-L. (1999) Follow up study of longstanding depression as a predictor of mortality in elderly people living in the community. *British Medical Journal* **318**: 432–433.

The table comes from a paper which examines the effect of depression upon mortality in elderly people. The authors assembled a cohort consisting of all people aged over 61 years living in Ahtari, Finland on January 1st 1984. Physical health and functional abilities were determined by a general practitioner, and depression was diagnosed according to DSM–III criteria after a semi-structured interview. At a follow up interview in 1989–90, 94% of the original cohort was re-interviewed. On the basis of the two interviews, people were described as: depressed at both interviews (*n*=78); depressed in 1984 but not at follow up (*n*=101); not depressed at either interview (*n*=634).

Mortality up to December 31st 1995 was determined from official statistics. Predictors of mortality are summarised in the table:

Predictors of mortality according to Cox's model: this adjusts for multiple associations

Variable	Relative risk (95% CI)
High age (continuous variable)	1.1 (1.07 to 1.12)
Male sex	1.4 (1.04 to 1.80)
Smoking	1.7 (1.11 to 2.70)
Lowered functional abilities*	1.7 (1.21 to 2.39)
Poor physical health**	1.8 (1.38 to 2.42)
Depression***	
first interview only	1.3 (0.85 to 1.87)
both interviews	1.5 (1.06 to 2.20)

*reference group, fully functionally independent subjects.
**reference group, subjects reported in good physical health by general practitioner.
***reference group, subjects who were not depressed at either interview.

Question B1

(a)   Why did the authors examine the effects of physical health on mortality, if their interest was in the effects of depression?

[4 marks]

(b)   Name three other variables of this type that it would have been relevant to measure.

[2 marks each up to a maximum of 6 marks]

Question B2

(a)   What does the table show overall,

[2 marks]

and specifically regarding depression?

[2 marks]

(b)   Were lowered functional abilities independently associated with mortality? Explain your reasoning.

[4 marks]

(c)   What important data regarding mortality and depression have not been presented here?

[2 marks]

Question B3

(a)   What implications (if any) does this study have regarding clinical practice in psychiatry?

[4 marks]

(b)   Give four limitations of the design and execution of this study.

[I mark each up to a maximum of 4 marks]

(c)   What does the study demonstrate regarding the effects of treating depression on mortality?

[2 marks]

Model answers by Helen Kenny

Question Al

(a)
The randomisation process ensures that all subjects entering into this study have an equal chance of being allocated to any of the treatment groups, be it the three-way or two-way groups. Its main purpose is to eliminate bias, which occurs when experimenters are allowed to influence subject allocation. The presence of potential confounding factors becomes equally likely in each group and, hence, the groups are balanced for important prognostic factors that might affect the therapeutic outcome, e.g. age, gender, symptom severity and duration, etc.

(b)
Preference randomisation permits the assessment of the effects of patient choice on treatment efficacy, by attempting to minimise bias introduced by any difference in baseline patient expectation and motivation.

(c)
Block randomisation was used to assure equal numbers in each treatment arm at any stage in the study, as recruitment of sufficient subjects needed to ensure the study had sufficient power was a lengthy process.

Only the three-way randomised group data are given in the paper. These show comparable numbers in each treatment group, albeit the cognitive–behavioural therapy (CBT) group was two patients short of the required 65 needed to ensure sufficient study power.

(d)
Stratified randomisation was used to ensure proportionate representation of subjects scoring high or low on the BDI in each treatment group.

The baseline BDI score was considered to be one of the most important factors influencing response to treatment, as it is a marker of symptom severity. Without stratified randomisation of subjects bias might have been introduced, in the form of a confounding variable, if the treatment groups had varied in the proportion of high and low scorers. This was particularly important, as the BDI was the only clinical outcome measure used.

Question A2

(a)
(i)   Increased
(ii) Decreased
(iii) Decreased

(b)
A power calculation is used to determine how many subjects are needed for a clinical trial to have a good chance of detecting a clinically significant difference on a particular outcome variable, assuming that a real difference does exist. It minimises the chance of a Type II error occurring (i.e. a false-negative result). The 90% power of this study means that you have a 90% chance of detecting a mean difference in outcome between the groups of 3.5 (SD 8) points on the BDI, when such a difference is truly present. To achieve a significant level of 5%, 65 subjects are required in each treatment group.

(c)
There is much greater variability in the data on costs than in the BDI scores, among the three treatment groups, as evidenced by the higher standard deviations about the mean. One reason for this is that the BDI is a unitary standardised measure, with definite end-points, whereas the cost data relies on a number of different measures, all of which are highly variable. This was particularly evident in the spread of indirect costs. This may indicate that the sample size was too small to detect differences in cost, as the power calculation was made on the basis of expected clinical outcomes.

Question A3

(a)
1.   At 12 months, all treatment modalities (CBT, non-directive counselling, usual GP care) appeared equally effective at reducing depressive symptoms, as evidenced by a reduction in the BDI scores.

2.   From baseline to 4 months, there was a statistically significant change in BDI scores between the three groups ($p = 0.008$), with the two therapy groups showing a greater reduction in BDI scores, and hence depressive symptoms in the short term, when compared with the usual GP care group.

3.   From 4 months to 12 months, there was a further statistically significant change in BDI scores between the three groups ($p = 0.006$), with the usual GP care group appearing to show more change than the other two groups.

(b)

No.

The results show a statistically significant difference between the three groups in the reduction of BDI scores from baseline to 4 months ($p = 0.008$). This appears to be most pronounced for the two therapy groups (CBT and counselling). However, there is no evidence of a statistical comparison having been performed between the CBT group and the usual GP care group.

Question A4

(a)

Cost-effectiveness analysis.

(b)

A cost-effectiveness analysis measures the net cost of providing a service as well as the outcomes obtained. Outcomes are reported in a single unit of measurement. In this study, the clinical outcome measure (the BDI score) highlighted the difference between treatment groups in the short versus long term. The costs (direct and indirect) incurred by each group were then calculated in monetary terms.

(c)

1.   A cost–benefit analysis assesses whether the cost of an intervention is worth the benefit, by measuring both in the same units, usually monetary. This was not attempted in this study.

2.   A cost–utility analysis converts effects into personal preferences (or utilities) and describes how much it costs for some additional quality gain (e.g. cost per additional quality-adjusted life-year, or QALY). No such conversion was made in this study.

3.   A cost-minimisation analysis assumes that the health benefits of each intervention are equal, and hence only costs are analysed, and the least costly alternative is chosen. This study assessed both clinical effectiveness and cost-effectiveness, and highlights differences in the rate of clinical effect.

Question A5

(a)

Discounting describes a process where present cost valuations are reduced according to a specified discount rate over time. This allows for the effects of uncertainty when calculating the costs and benefits of future events, where the value people place on these can vary according to time. Costs obtained after discounting represent the current worth of future events.

Discounting was not considered necessary in this study as neither costs nor benefits were recorded beyond 12 months. In the UK, the discount rate for costs is a set percentage per annum.

(b)

Production losses were calculated from information gathered directly from subjects, and addressed lost earnings. As such, this was not externally validated. This approach also values the health of professional people higher than that of manual workers, homemakers, or the unemployed. It might have been preferable to derive the cost of sick days from the average national wage. Other indirect production costs, such as spouse/carer time off work, were not included.

(c)

(i)   At 4 months, there appears to be minimal difference between the three groups in respect of direct, indirect and total costs. The slight increase in costs for the non-directive counselling group, and the slight reduction for the CBT group, when compared with the usual GP care group, cannot be interpreted without statistical analysis being provided. What is evident is the large variation in costing for each group, with large standard deviations and confidence intervals, which suggests that the results are not statistically significant.

(ii)   At 12 months the costs are higher, but again there is minimal difference between the groups for direct, indirect and total costs. The degree of data spread suggests that any difference is not significant as the confidence intervals are wide and span zero.

Question A6

(a)

The purpose of the sensitivity analysis was to increase the validity of the economic analysis results. It evaluates the robustness of the results to changes in certain parameters, to test the consistency of the results over a range of assumptions. This study looked at how sensitive the results were to using full costs of missed appointments, use of the most expensive medications and using the national average wage as opposed to self-reported wages.

(b)

Table A3 shows that there is no significant difference in the total costs between the three groups at 12 months. The p value of 0.63 shows that there is a 63% chance that any difference seen is produced by chance. In this study, a p value of 5% was accepted as a marker of statistical significance, and the threshold below which the null hypothesis would be discounted. It also shows that the differences in total cost, when each of the three sensitivity analyses was applied, remained non-significant.

(c)

(i)   The main disadvantage of univariate sensitivity analysis is that only one parameter can be changed at a time. Multivariate analysis allows for the values of two or more sets of parameters to be changed simultaneously, and hence is a more advanced test of how robust the results are in the real world.

(ii)   In Table A3, only three parameters were altered. How robust the results are to change in other areas cannot be examined.

(d)

If therapists' salaries were increased, this may make it more likely that the direct costs in the two therapy groups will be significantly higher than usual GP care, and show the latter to be more cost-effective.

Question A7

(a)

Employing practice-based counsellors or cognitive–behavioural therapists for short term interventions may enable patients with moderately severe depression to recover more quickly in the short term (4 months) and be more cost-effective, but there is no evidence of cost-effectiveness when compared with usual GP care in the long term.

(b)

Dr Smith's practice is likely to differ from those of the study such that the findings may not be applicable.

1.   One reason is the potential differences in the patient population. The study population came from inner city areas in England, whereas Dr Smith serves an area in rural Scotland. They may differ in terms of incidence of depression, symptom severity, comorbidity, coping strategies, psychological mindedness and willingness to consider psychological therapies, etc.

2.   Dr Smith may not have ready access to suitably qualified and experienced counsellors and psychologists, willing to provide a practice-based intervention for up to 12 sessions. Extra cost may be needed to employ or contract in these services, and geographical factors may mitigate against regular contact.

3.   Dr Smith's usual care of patients with depression may differ from that of the GPs in the study. As a single-handed GP in a rural area, he may not be as up-to-date with current treatment strategies, or have the time to apply them. Alternatively, he may be attuned to the needs of his population, and the continuity of care afforded may make him more effective at treating depression.

Question B1

(a)

Physical health is an important prognostic factor when looking at mortality as an outcome measure. It is an important confounding variable when studying the relationship between longstanding depression and mortality in elderly people, as the prevalence of physical health problems is higher. It is possible that patients in poorer health are more likely to experience depression as a result of the associated stress and disability. If this was not adjusted for, then a false association between longstanding depression and mortality may result. It is also possible that longstanding depression may have an adverse effect on physical health, and hence may itself be a predictor of early mortality – the hypothesis in this study.

(b)
Other relevant, potential confounding variables requiring measurement include the use of antidepressant medication, alcohol intake and social background (marital status, living arrangements/care required, etc.).

Question B2

(a)
The table shows that, in the cohort defined, those individuals exhibiting one of the variables outlined had an increased mortality risk, when compared with individuals without this variable (e.g. smokers versus non-smokers). The relative risks are not impressive however (less than 3). Although the narrow confidence intervals, which, except for depression at the first interview only, do not cross 1, suggest statistical significance, it is unlikely that this is of clinical significance.

The table shows that subjects who were shown to be depressed at both interviews were 1.5 times more likely than subjects who did not have depression at either interview to die in the time period of the study. Those with depression only at the first interview appeared to have a higher mortality risk, but this was not statistically significant, as evidenced by the wide confidence interval.

(b)
The table suggests that lowered functional capacity is an independent risk factor for dying during the course of this study, when compared with a reference group of fully functioning, independent subjects. It is unclear, however, how the researchers separated functional ability from physical health, which is listed as another independent variable. It is possible that those less functionally able are also those in poorer physical health. There are few details as to how the reference group was chosen, and whether they were matched for all variables except functional ability.

(c)
It would be important to give details of cause of death (suicide or physical causes) as well as timing of death in relation to age/depressive episode.

Question B3

(a)
The study's relevance to clinical practice lies in the cause of death, and how the depressive episodes were managed. Based on the information available, it could be concluded that longstanding depression in the elderly is a predictor of early mortality. If this is via increased susceptibility to physical illness, then the clinician and GP need to be more vigilant and monitor physical health. If suicide is a common cause of death, then risk assessment procedures need to be evaluated, and management options considered. The study appears to imply that a treated single episode of depression does not increase risk of early mortality, but untreated depression does. Whether this is due to the depression being untreated or unsuccessfully treated needs to be clarified. Relevant information such as use of antidepressant medication needs to be recorded.

(b)
Limitations of this study include:

1. The study population comprised a population of elderly people of different ages, backgrounds, physical and mental health. As such, this introduces a number of potential confounding variables, with no matched comparison group. An inception cohort may have been preferable, of similar subjects with similar depressive symptoms, with a comparison group of matched subjects free of depression.

2. The representativeness of the residents of Ahtari, Finland, needs to be considered, as the results may not generalise to other populations.

3. There is limited information documented on important factors such as severity of depression, past psychiatric history and treatment interventions. Whether this was documented is not known.

4. The issue of interviewer bias needs to be addressed by more information on who was involved in the diagnosis of depression and assessment of physical health and functional ability. Ideally, the assessment of depression should have been conducted by a separate interviewer, blind to the GP's assessment of physical health and functional ability.

(c)
The study results seem to suggest that successfully treated depression in the elderly does not increase mortality risk. In contrast, longstanding depression, presumably unsuccessfully treated, appears to be a predictor of early mortality. No information is provided, however, on whether those subjects with depression in the first interview were in fact treated for their depression, or whether natural resolution occurred. Symptom severity is also unknown.

MRCPsych Part II Examination
Critical Review Paper
Spring 2003

Please read the instructions carefully before going further.

Instructions

1. This examination lasts for 90 minutes.
2. The paper has TWO questions, Question A and Question B, *each of which should be answered using separate answer booklets as indicated.*
3. You must *attempt* ALL parts of BOTH questions.
4. A total of 100 marks has been allocated to the whole paper. Each part of each question is worth 10 marks. Therefore, Question A is worth 70 marks, and Question B is worth 30 marks.
5. In answering Question A, candidates may wish to glance briefly at the questions they are asked to answer (on pages 117–120 of the paper), before reading the details of the research (described on pages 114–117).
6. Where you give more than the requested number of answers, you will only be marked on that number, e.g. If you are asked for 5 examples and give 6, you will only be marked on the first 5.
7. Candidates are advised to bring a calculator to the examination hall for this paper. Candidates are only permitted to take a noiseless, cordless, pocket-sized non-programmable calculator WITHOUT printout or graphic/word display facilities.
8. Please do not remove this Examination paper from the Examination Room.

Question A

Psychiatric diagnosis versus impairment in young people

You are working in a child guidance clinic, which is attracting an increasing rate of new referrals, and is struggling with a growing waiting list. A recent audit of the clinic suggests that many of the patients treated at the clinic are not given a psychiatric diagnosis on discharge. This finding has led the main purchasers of the service to conclude that the clinic has too low a threshold for accepting cases and, if the threshold were raised to include only those children with clear psychiatric diagnoses, the waiting list could be cut considerably. You and your colleagues are worried that confining your work to those children who warrant a formal psychiatric diagnosis only after assessment will not serve the needs of the local community. You discuss your fears with one of the non-executive directors of the service (an accountant with no experience of clinical practice). This non-executive director, keen to learn more, asks the local medical librarian to find some literature to inform the discussion. The librarian finds the following paper:

Angold, A. *et al.* Impaired but undiagnosed. *J Am Acad Child Adolesc Psychiatry* 1999; **38**(2): 129–137.

Your consultant asks you to appraise the paper and to meet with the non-executive director to discuss your appraisal.

The paper

Background

This paper describes results from the Great Smoky Mountains Study, a longitudinal study among young people drawn from both rural and urban communities. A representative sample of 4500 young people, aged 9, 11 or 13 years, was drawn from the public school system in one state of the United States.

The researchers aimed to investigate the prevalence and outcomes of individuals with psychosocial impairment not meeting DSM−III−R criteria for any well-defined disorders.

Methods

Screening: A parent (usually the child's mother) was asked to complete a screening questionnaire, which used a subset of 55 questions from the Child Behaviour Checklist, a well validated and reliable 138-item scale used to assess symptoms, behaviour and social competence in children and adolescents.

Recruitment: Recruited into the study were (a) all young people with scores above a pre-defined threshold on the screening questionnaire and (b) a random 1:10 sample of the remaining eligible children. As the sample was selected on the basis of a screening questionnaire, to produce unbiased general population parameter estimates it was necessary to weight the analyses. The initial weights were, therefore, the inverse of the sampling fractions from each screen stratum. These initial weights were then corrected for age, group and gender.

Procedure: Two sets of interviews were carried out, 1 year apart. From the initial sample of 1015 subjects, 913 (90%) were successfully followed up. Separate interviews were conducted with the children enrolled into the study and, as far as possible, with one of their parents. Of the primary caretakers interviewed,

84% were biological mothers, and 7% were biological fathers, the remainder were carers in close contact with the child.

Assessment measures: The baseline interview included three assessment instruments, all with established validity and reliability. For all three instruments, the questions referred to the 3 months preceding the interview.

(a)   *Child and Adolescent Psychiatric Assessment (CAPA)*. This elicits symptoms and impairment in 17 areas of functioning. The schedule has been found to identify whether or not any impairment found is attributable to symptoms, or whether this is due purely to relationship problems. Following this assessment a diagnosis is made or not according to DSM–III–R, the extent of impairment in social functioning determined and how far this is related to difficulties in relationships.

(b)   *Child and Adolescent Burden Assessment (CABA)*. Completed by parents after the CAPA, this measures the extent to which burdens perceived by the parents are caused by, or exacerbated by, their child's emotional or behavioural difficulties.

(c)   *Child and Adolescent Services Assessment (CASA)*. This assesses the specialist contact which the child has had for its psychiatric or behavioural problems, in a wide variety of settings (mental health services, school, etc.).

Once an impairment had been determined to be present according to the rules set out in the CAPA glossary, interviewers were required to question the participants about what aspects of their symptomatology had led to that impairment. In the case of impairments in human relationships, it was possible to code a "pure" impairment unrelated to symptoms of psychiatric disorders. A child might have had both longstanding oppositional behaviours and a more recent onset of depressive symptoms and also might have reported a serious problem in his/her sibling relationships. The interviewer would collect information about whether the oppositional behaviour had contributed to the sibling relationship problems and find out whether the appearance of depression had affected these. For example, if the child reported that his/her failure to comply with the rules of games and tendency to get angry in interactions had led to problems with siblings, but that there had been no change in these difficulties since he/she had been depressed, an impairment in sibling relationships only would be coded. On the other hand, if the depression had led to increased irritability and withdrawal from siblings, an impairment due to depressive symptoms would be coded.

Results from the CAPA, CABA and CASA were used to divide the sample into five subgroups at baseline:

(A)   subjects with neither DSM–III–R, psychiatric diagnosis nor impairment (*No diagnosis or impairment*);

(B)   those with a DSM–III–R, diagnosis but no impairment (*Diagnosis only*);

(C)   those with impairment attributable to purely relationship problems, coded as V codes in DSM–III–R (*Relationship impairment*).

(D)   those with impairment due to symptoms but insufficient to fulfil a formal DSM–III–R, diagnosis (*Symptomatic impairment*);

(E)   those with both psychiatric diagnosis and impairment (*Diagnosis + impairment*)

The authors wished to determine which young people reached the criteria for 'caseness' at follow-up

A child in the study was defined as a 'case' if he or she fulfilled any one of the following criteria:

(1)   Receipt of help from specialist mental health services;

(2)   Receipt of help from school-based mental health services;

(3)   Perceived as a burden by the parent;

(4)   Appraisal by parent or child that the child had a problem;

(5)   Appraisal by parent or child that the child needed specialist mental health help.

Analysis: The analyses relevant to this extract of the paper aimed to test two hypotheses:

(i) At baseline, the numbers of young people categorised in individual subgroups B to E would be present in increased frequency amongst those children in contact with specialist mental health services compared with the remainder of the sample.

(ii) 'Caseness' at follow-up would not be accurately predicted by psychiatric diagnosis (with or without impairment) at baseline. The authors hypothesised that, even among those children who did not warrant a DSM–III–R diagnosis at baseline, some of those with impairments would qualify as 'cases' at follow-up.

Results

The authors first investigated whether the five subgroups above were equally prevalent among those using specialist mental health services and those not using these services in the 3 months prior to the first interview. These results are shown in Table I.

Table I. Weighted percentage frequencies of the five subgroups among Mental Health Service Users versus Non-Users at initial assessment

	Subgroup				
	A	B	C	D	E
	No diagnosis or impairment	Diagnosis only	Relationship impairment	Symptomatic impairment	Diagnosis plus impairment
% MHS Non-Users[a]	68	12	5	9	6
% MHS Users[b]	27	9	4	21	38
Odds ratio	0.2	0.8	0.9	2.8	9.5
95% CI[c]	0.1 to 0.4	0.4 to 1.7	0.3 to 2.4	1.1 to 6.9	4.3 to 21.1

[a] Children who were not in contact with specialist mental health services at initial assessment (N = 933) (contact data missing on 2 children)
[b] Children who were in contact with specialist mental health services at initial assessment (N = 80)
[c] 95% confidence interval of the odds ratio

The authors then examined the outcomes at 1-year follow up of the five different subgroups above. Within each subgroup, they measured the percentage of children who at 1-year follow-up fulfilled at least one of the five 'caseness' criteria. These results are shown in Table 2 (column I).

Column II in Table 2 presents another way of classifying outcomes for patients in each of the five subgroups. Column II shows, for each of the subgroups A–E identified at baseline, the percentage of children in contact with specialist mental health services at follow-up.

Table 2. Breakdown by subgroup (A to E) of percentage of 'cases' (column I) and percentage of patients in contact with Specialist Mental Health Services (column II) in the general population at follow-up

		Column (columns I and II will be referred to in the questions below)	
	Subgroup	I % "Cases" at follow-up	II % Patients in each Subgroup (A–E) in contact with Mental Health Services at follow-up
A	No diagnosis or impairment	35%	2%
B	Diagnosis only	76%	6%
C	Relationship impairment	87%	3%
D	Symptomatic impairment	75%[a]	16%[p]
E	Diagnosis + impairment	96%[a,b]	18%[q]

[a] All these frequencies are significantly greater (p < 0.05) than in Subgroup A
[b] This is significantly greater (P < 0.05) than the frequencies in Subgroups B, C or D

[p] This is greater (p < 0.05) than frequencies for subgroups A and C, but no different from subgroup E
[q] This is greater (p < 0.05) than frequencies for subgroups A, B and C

The authors' main conclusion is that children and adolescents, who do not meet DSM−III−R diagnostic criteria for any well-defined disorder but show symptoms plus psychosocial impairment, have enduring problems and should be regarded as suffering from a psychiatric disorder.

Question AI

(a)   What type of study is this?

[1 mark]

    Give two reasons to explain your answer

[2 marks each up to a maximum of 4 marks]

(b)   Was the sample in this study an inception cohort?

[1 mark]

    Justify your answer.

[4 marks]

Question A2

List five strengths of the *design* of this study (make sure you distinguish between design strengths and other features, which are associated with the *execution* of the study).

[2 marks for each feature up to a maximum of 10 marks]

Question A3

(a)   Describe three main findings comparing users of specialist mental health services (MHS Users) with those who were not in contact with such services (MHS Non-Users).

[6 marks]

(b)   The authors indicate that they "weighted" the analyses that they carried out that are indicated in the Tables. Explain briefly what weighting means in this context.

[2 marks]

Why did the authors do this? Explain your answers carefully.

[2 marks]

Question A4

You wish to know how good "having been allocated a diagnosis" is as a test to predict "caseness" in a year's time. For this question, assume that "caseness" at follow-up is the gold standard, and the presence or absence of a diagnosis is the test. In other words, subjects in subgroups B and E are equivalent to a "positive" test, while subjects in subgroups A, C, and D are equivalent to a "negative" test.

From the information in the original paper, you estimated the numbers of young people (amongst the 1,013 people studied) who would have become "a case" in a year, both in those initially allocated and those not allocated a diagnosis. (N.B. You may assume that these figures are correct and use them in your calculations. Do NOT try to verify them.)

No. of subjects in categories B and E who would become "a case" at 1 year: 243

No. of subjects in categories A, C and D who would become "a case" at 1 year: 354

Total number of subjects in categories B and E: 283

Total number of subjects in categories A, C and D: 730

(a)   Construct a 2×2 table to calculate measures for the usefulness of this test.

[6 marks]

(b)   From the table that you have constructed calculate the following measures for the test in the study population (to the nearest %):

(i)   Sensitivity

[2 marks]

(ii)   Specificity

[2 marks]

Question A5

(a)   From your answers in question A4, calculate

(i)   the likelihood ratio for a positive test result.

[I mark]

(ii)   the likelihood ratio for a negative test result.

[I mark]

(b)   Compare the sensitivity and specificity and explain what these results mean.

[2 marks]

What do the two likelihood ratios indicate?

[2 marks]

(c)   What are the implications of allocation of a diagnosis and non-allocation of a diagnosis for a young person in relationship to reaching the criteria for caseness one year subsequently?

[4 marks]

Question A6

(a)   Among those who show neither symptomatology nor impairment (Subgroup A) at baseline, 35% of them score as "cases" within a year. This appears an excessively high rate of "caseness". Give three possible explanations for such high percentage?

[2 marks for each up to a maximum of 6 marks]

(b)   From Table 2 87% of those who showed a relationship impairment (but no significant psychiatric symptomatology) at follow-up were "cases", yet only 3% were in contact with Mental Health Services. Give two reasons from the information given in the paper which might account for this discrepancy?

[2 marks for each up to a maximum of 4 marks]

Question A7

(a)   How would you *summarise and interpret* the results in column I of Table 2 for the non-executive director? Give 2 important findings from the Table. Remember that as an accountant he can read the figures just as you can (so do not simply put the results into words); he requires an appropriate interpretation. This may require you to indicate the meaning of the results in the context of what you have learned about the methods.

[4 marks]

(b)   How would you explain to the non-executive director the relevance of this paper and its findings to the original query about whether diagnosis was important in this area? Give 3 main findings.

[2 marks for each up to a maximum of 6 marks]

Question B

The following figure is taken from a paper which reported a research study undertaken in Sweden that examined the association between use of cardiovascular drugs and suicide (Lindberg G *et al*. Use of calcium channel blockers and risk of suicide: ecological findings confirmed in a population based cohort study. *British Medical Journal* 1998: 316 (7 March).

The authors estimated rates of use of various drugs by obtaining dispensing rates from pharmacies, and suicide rates from standard national data. The study was conducted in 152 municipalities in Sweden, and the figure shows the relation between use of calcium channel-blockers and suicide rate in each of those municipalities.

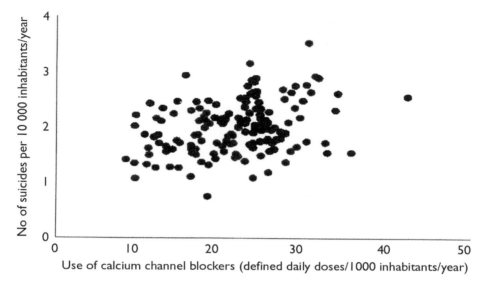

Question B1

(a)   Describe what the figure shows.

[4 marks]

(b)   What statistical test would you expect the authors to have applied to the data presented in the figure?

[6 marks]

Question B2

(a)   The authors discuss the possibility that *confounding* might explain their findings. What does this term mean?

[4 mark]

(b)   Give two examples of possible confounders in this study and explain your choice.

[1 mark for each confounder and 2 marks for each explanation up to a maximum of 6 marks]

Question B3

Studies of this sort, which compare the characteristics of whole populations, are sometimes called *ecological studies*.

(a) Name a key disadvantage of this study design.

[2 marks]

(b) Give two other designs that might be used to answer the question?

[2 marks for each up to a maximum of 4 marks]

(c) Does this paper show that calcium channel blockers lead to an increased risk of suicide? Explain your reasoning.

[4 marks]

Model answers by Danny H. Sullivan

Question A1

(a)

This is a cohort study. The sample is a representative group of young people, all of whom have been screened for caseness. The design of this study is prospective, relying on interviews one year apart. Thus, the cohort have been examined for exposure (caseness) and followed up for development of problems over time. The longitudinal design is critical for a cohort study.

(b)

This is not an inception cohort. The group initially screened has been further selected. Those who have scores above a threshold, and a 1:10 random sample of the other children, are the study group. If this were an inception cohort, all of the initial group would be followed up, rather than the selected group. To compensate for this selection, the authors have weighted the analyses.

Question A2

(a)

Design strengths are:

1. The study incorporates a large sample, increasing the power of the study and thus maximising the likelihood that the results are statistically significant.

2. Data have been collected from multiple sources – usually parents and their children – to increase the likelihood of detecting symptoms or impairment. Consequently the rates of disorder are more likely to reflect actual problems than either dataset alone.

3. The sample appears representative – that is, it covers multiple age groups, both urban and rural, and incorporates those with problems as well as those without, reducing and accommodating selection bias.

4. The measures used are reliable and validated in these populations. Thus, screening of the populations is likely to detect cases.

5. A prospective design reduces the likelihood of ascertainment bias and other systematic deviations. Rather than relying on retrospective methodology, the study is able to correlate variables at entry with outcomes at one year.

Question A3

(a)

1. Those who have both a clinical diagnosis and symptomatic impairment are much more likely to use mental health services than any other group.

2. Children who exhibit symptomatic impairment but do not fulfil criteria sufficient to meet DSM–III–R diagnosis are still significantly more likely to be in contact with mental health services.

3. Children who have neither a clinical diagnosis nor symptomatic impairment are significantly less likely to be in contact with mental health services.

(b)

The sample is stratified and thus weighting ensures that each stratum is represented proportionately. Weighting is an adjustment which compensates for selection bias. The use of a screening questionnaire to enrol subjects will include more cases than occur randomly. Weighting will result in the data more closely reflecting population norms.

Weighting corrects the error of selecting from screened populations, which would otherwise result in systematic deviations towards pathology. Without weighting, the sample would appear more likely to exhibit diagnoses and impairment, as the selected group would skew data. It ensures that the samples from each stratum are representative of the population from which they are drawn.

Question A4

(a)

	caseness at I year	non-caseness at I year	Total
diagnosis positive (B + E)	243	40	283
diagnosis negative (A + C + D)	354	376	730
Total	597	416	1013

(b)

(i) Sensitivity = 254/597
     = 0.42

(ii) Specificity = 376/416
     = 0.90

Question A5

(a)

(i) LR^+ = sensitivity/(1 − specificity)
         = 0.42/0.10
         = 4.2

(ii) LR^- = (1 − sensitivity)/specificity
         = 0.58/0.90
         = 0.64

(b)

Sensitivity refers to the proportion of people who become cases at one year, who have a diagnosis. Specificity refers to the proportion of those who do not become cases who do not have a diagnosis – the true negatives. In this case, these two measures reflect the accuracy of a diagnosis in determining who will be a case at one year. Low sensitivity here suggests that a diagnosis does not predict very well who will be a case. However, the high specificity in this sample indicates that those without diagnoses are not very likely to be cases at one year.

The two likelihood ratios indicate that a diagnosis is suggestive of contact with mental health services at one year; and that lack of diagnosis correlates with not being in contact with mental health services, although not as strongly.

(c)

If allocated a diagnosis, it is more likely that the subject will be in contact with mental health services at follow-up. However, those without diagnoses who exhibit relational or symptomatic impairment are also more likely to be in contact with mental health services. In fact, the rates of those with a diagnosis (24%) and those without (21%) are not greatly different. Thus, allocation of a diagnosis does not correlate strongly with ongoing mental health caseness.

Question A6

(a)

1. This is a selected sample. Entry relied on scoring above a predefined threshold on the screening questionnaire (the Child Behaviour Checklist). Thus, even if there is no diagnosis or impairment at baseline, many children may require relatively little change to reach caseness.

2. The ages at which subjects are studied – 9, 11 and 13 years – occur in a period that may include developmental and situational changes. Transition into teenage years may have been associated with increased conflict or the development of psychiatric symptomatology related to these transitions.

3. The definition of caseness is a broad one. It includes contact with services, appraisal that there is a problem or parental description of the child as a burden. Enrolment in the study may have alerted the family to service options and increased referral bias, or at least awareness of services.

(b)

1.   The definition of caseness might include a number of situations which would not necessarily result in contact with mental health services. For instance, parental perception of the child as a burden might indicate relationship impairment but would not necessarily result in contact with services.

2.   Relational problems such as bullying or sibling rivalry would qualify as caseness but are more likely to be dealt with informally or in school; it would be unusual for these children to be in contact with mental health services. This reflects the broad definition used here for caseness.

Question A7

(a)

The results show that those assessed at baseline as having both diagnosis and impairment are most likely to have problems at follow-up (almost all children); and that those with no diagnosis and impairment at baseline are less likely to. What is surprising, however, is that those who showed either diagnosis or impairment were significantly more likely to be cases at follow-up – over three-quarters of each category. This means that children who do not qualify for a diagnosis, but have impairment, are likely to have future problems sufficient to warrant attention.

(b)

1.   These results show that a narrow reliance on diagnosis and impairment alone as criteria for admission into a mental health service will miss significant numbers of children who have problems. Although these problems do not register on operationalised diagnostic criteria, they are clinically significant and warrant attention.

2.   Also noticeable is that children with symptomatic impairment (but no diagnosis) are almost as likely as those with both diagnosis and impairment to be in contact with services. This suggests that services select patients not on the basis of diagnosis, but rather on that of symptomatic impairment.

3.   It is also conspicuous that, despite registering highly as cases, those with relational impairment alone were very unlikely to be in contact with services at follow-up. These children seem not to be identified as warranting service input and it may be that their symptoms are attributed to relational problems rather than psychopathology. Nevertheless, their problems seem significant and they are not receiving services. This is an area of unmet need.

Question B1

(a)

This is a scatter diagram. It compares the suicide rate with the rate of calcium channel blocker use. The trend of data suggests a positive correlation. That is, greater use of calcium channel blockers appears to be associated with an increased suicide rate. The correlation is reasonably strong.

(b)

The authors should have applied a test of correlation. This measures the degree of association between two observations. In this case, there appears to be a positive correlation between the rate of suicide and the rate of calcium channel blocker use. As both variables will likely have a normal distribution, Pearson's correlation coefficient can be used; if one or both observations is distributed otherwise, Spearman's rank correlation coefficient can be used.

Question B2

(a)

Confounding refers to the possibility that there are other independent factors which might account for the association. Unlike bias, these factors are alternative relationships between the exposure (use of calcium channel blockers) and the outcome (suicide). They are on the same causal pathway, and may be an independent risk factor or a protective factor. Confounders are only important if they differ between study groups.

(b)

1.   Cardiovascular disease may cause or lead to depression. If this happens, the drug prescribed may not cause suicide; rather, the underlying disease would be the causal factor. If this were the case, *all* cardiovascular drugs would show an increase in suicide rates.

2.   The preponderance of men who suffer cardiovascular disease, along with the known elevated incidence of male suicide compared with female suicide, might account for the increase. Thus, prescription of calcium channel blockers, elevated in men, would be a proxy for male gender, and men are already known to be more likely to commit suicide.

Question B3

(a)
Ecological studies may suggest associations, but cannot prove causality. Other variables, not taken into account, may be responsible for the association between exposure and outcome.

(b)
Alternative study designs might demonstrate this link. A *case–control* study might show significant differences in suicide rates between those on calcium channel blockers and those not on these medications. Another possibility is a *clinical trial* comparing these drugs against other drugs, using suicide rates as an endpoint, rather than blood pressure or other variables.

(c)
This paper demonstrates an association between calcium channel blocker use and suicide. Although there may be a causal link, there are a number of confounders and it is therefore difficult to claim that the drugs lead to an increased risk of suicide. It may be that the population prescribed the drugs is already at increased risk owing to depression or other independent variables; or that prescribers select these drugs for depressed patients. Although the association seems to be present, it is not necessarily causal.

MRCPsych Part II Examination
Critical Review Paper
Autumn 2003

Please read the instructions carefully before going further.

Instructions

1. This examination lasts for 90 minutes.
2. The paper has TWO questions, Question A and Question B, *each of which should be answered using separate answer booklets as indicated.*
3. You must *attempt* ALL parts of BOTH questions.
4. A total of 100 marks has been allocated to the whole paper. Each part of each question is worth 10 marks. Therefore, Question A is worth 70 marks, and Question B is worth 30 marks.
5. In answering Question A, candidates may wish to glance briefly at the questions they are asked to answer (on pages 129–131 of the paper), before reading the details of the research (described on pages 128–129).
6. Where you give more than the requested number of answers, you will only be marked on that number, e.g. If you are asked for 5 examples and give 6, you will only be marked on the first 5.
7. Candidates are advised to bring a calculator to the examination hall for this paper. Candidates are only permitted to take a noiseless, cordless, pocket-sized non-programmable calculator WITHOUT printout or graphic/word display facilities.
8. Please do not remove this Examination paper from the Examination Room.

Question A

Cognitive therapy and recovery from acute psychosis

You are a consultant in general adult psychiatry with a busy practice. You are responsible for numerous patients with schizophrenia and arrange several acute admissions for relapse per week. The team psychologist has recently been trained in the application of cognitive behavioural therapy for psychosis as part of the work with the assertive outreach team. You, however, were impressed by the publication of Drury et al., B. J. Psych 1996, which you believe demonstrated that CBT improved psychotic symptoms and recovery time in acute relapse. You therefore approach the Trust mental health manager with the request that the psychologist develop an acute inpatient CBT practice in preference to assertive outreach.

The manager refers you to the publication below:

Cognitive therapy and recovery from acute psychosis: a controlled trial. 3. Five-year follow-up. Drury, V., Birchwood, M. and Cochrane, R. *British Journal of Psychiatry* (2000) **177**, 8–14.

Summary of study

62 hospitalised acutely psychotic patients were randomised to one of two groups: cognitive therapy, or recreational activities with informal support, using a stratified sampling technique. Of 117 acute patients screened, 62 fulfilled inclusion criteria and were entered into the trial, but 10 patients allocated to cognitive therapy and 12 to recreational activities dropped out. 40 patients therefore completed the treatment phase of the study.

Both groups received a mean of 8 hours per week therapist contact time for a maximum of six months. The cognitive therapy was delivered in four stages over the course of recovery: individual therapy, group therapy, family psychoeducation and support, and skills groups/creative therapies. At baseline, the two groups did not differ on any relevant clinical factor. Nine months after treatment began, only 5% of the cognitive therapy group, versus 56% of the recreational activities group, showed moderate or severe residual symptoms. These assessments were not blind to treatment group status.

Patients were followed up five years later: 17 in each group were available. They were assessed using four of the measures used for assessment at entry into the study.

Outcome measures included rating scales for positive symptoms, belief in delusions, insight and attitudes towards illness. Information on compliance, readmission and relapse not resulting in readmission was also available. Only data on relapse and readmission were compiled blindly.

Patients who had dropped out did not differ clinically from the rest.

Table I. Clinical course of groups at follow-up

	Cognitive therapy n = 17	Recreation/informal support n = 17
Mean no. of relapses (s.d.)	1.4 (1.6)	1.2 (1.4)
Mean no. of admissions (s.d.)	1.2 (1.4)	1.2 (1.4)
Median time in acute care (days)	26.5	32
Median time to first relapse (days)	821	345

There were no statistically significant between-group differences.

The authors reported their outcome variable analysis of variance (ANCOVA) for comparisons between the treatment groups at follow-up. The covariate was the corresponding baseline variable score. They examined their outcome variables for the whole sample, and also for the subgroup of patients who had not relapsed or who had relapsed only once.

Table 2. Outcome variables for whole groups, and subgroups with <1 relapse

Variable	Cognitive therapy		Recreational/informal		
	n	mean (s.d.)	n	support mean (s.d.)	p
Positive symptoms	16	1.9 (2.5)	17	3.2 (3.2)	0.055
Subgroup ≤1 relapse	10	0.8 (1.4)	12	3.8 (3.3)	0.002
Delusional beliefs	17	0.9 (2.0)	17	1.8 (2.2)	NS
Subgroup ≤1 relapse	10	0.1 (0.3)	12	2.2 (2.5)	0.022
Attitude to control over illness	15	7.5 (2.4)	16	9.4 (1.0)	0.007
Subgroup ≤1 relapse	10	7.3 (2.0)	11	9.3 (0.8)	0.012
Awareness of stigma	15	6.2 (1.5)	16	7.3 (1.4)	NS
Subgroup ≤1 relapse	10	6.0 (1.7)	11	7.4 (1.3)	0.056

All ratings scales are structured so that greater scores indicate greater problems.

Question A1

(a)   Considering its nature and timing and how the results were reported, give one advantage and one disadvantage of *each* of the following two aspects of follow-up assessment

(i)   consisting of a single rather than repeated assessments
(ii)   occurring five years later rather than at an earlier time.

[2 marks for each advantage and 2 marks for each disadvantage, up to a maximum of 8 marks]

(b)   Give one *other* advantage OR disadvantage of the follow-up assessments unrelated to the two aspects outlined in part (a) above.

[2 marks]

Question A2

(a)   State two advantages of the design and execution and analysis of this study, *excluding* matters relating to follow-up assessments.

(b)   State eight disadvantages of the design and execution and analysis of this study, *excluding* matters relating to follow-up assessments.

[1 mark each, up to a maximum of 10 marks]

Question A3

Examine Table I.

(a)   What are the four main findings regarding clinical course?

[I mark each, up to a maximum of 4 marks]

(b)   Is it likely that these data on numbers of relapses and readmissions are normally distributed? Explain your reasoning.

[3 marks]

(c)   Give three comments on the results for median time to first relapse, and any clinical implications.

[I mark each, up to a maximum of 3 marks]

Question A4

Examine Table 2.

(a)   What are the two main findings regarding outcome in the whole group?

[I mark each, up to a maximum of 2 marks]

(b)   How do the subgroup findings compare generally?

[2 marks]

(c)   Give one potential problem of a subgroup analysis.

[2 marks]

(d)   Six patients did not return their rating scales on delusions. The authors decided to allocate the maximum score on delusions to these patients when they carried out the analysis. Why did they do this?

[2 marks]

(e)   What would the authors have done, had they wanted to carry out a 'worst possible scenario' analysis?

[2 marks]

Question A5

(a)   You are unfamiliar with the rating scales used in this study. Identify any two pieces of information which you need to interpret the scores.

[I mark each up to a maximum of 2 marks]

(b)   Do statistically significant differences, represent clinical relevance? Give two reasons.

[2 marks for correct answer, I mark for each reason, up to a maximum of 4 marks]

(c)   This study could have reported numbers of 'responders' in groups rather than reporting differences between group means. Give two operational definitions of 'response' which could have been utilised in this study. Give one advantage and one disadvantage of this method.

[I mark for each definition, I for each advantage and disadvantage up to a maximum of 4 marks]

Question A6

(a)   How many patients per week would a full-time psychologist (who spent 40 hours per week seeing patients) be able to see if employed on the active intervention arm in this study?

[2 marks]

(b)   On average you admit five acutely psychotic patients per week and they stay an average of three weeks. What is the rolling total of patients (one mark) and what proportion of the patients could be taken on for CBT? (one mark)

[2 marks]

(c)   Give three ways to make this treatment more widely available in your service.

[2 marks each, up to a maximum of 6 marks]

Question A7

(a)   List five points which the manager might raise to support his or her argument that this study may not be applicable to the Trust.

[I mark each, up to a maximum of 5 marks]

(b)   Suppose the manager agrees to the psychologist working with inpatients as requested, and allocates you half a day a week of 'audit clerk' time (but nothing else) for the next three years to evaluate the effectiveness of this new service development. List five ways in which the audit clerk could evaluate the new service over the next three years.

[I mark each, up to a maximum of 5 marks]

Question B

Dothiepin

As a consultant psychiatrist, you saw a 59-year-old patient with depression and you considered prescribing dothiepin. However, your SHO was worried about the risk of ischaemic heart disease and drew your attention to the following paper:

Hippisley-Cox, J. *et al.* Antidepressants as risk factor for ischaemic heart disease: case–control study in primary care. *BMJ* 2001, **323**: 666–669.

Patients from 9 general practices between 1995–1999 who had a diagnosis of ischaemic heart disease were identified from computer records. For each of these patients identified, 4 to 6 controls without a recorded diagnosis of ischaemic heart disease, matched for age and sex, were selected by finding the patients closest in age from an ordered list of patients currently registered with the same practice. For both groups of patients, data on relevant clinical information and antidepressants prescribed were extracted. There were a total of 933 cases and 5,516 controls.

Table 1. Unadjusted and adjusted odds ratios

	Unadjusted odds ratio (95% CI)	Adjusted odds ratio* (95% CI)
SSRI ever	1.55 (1.18 to 2.01)	1.29 (0.89 to 1.87)
Tricyclic antidepressants ever	1.67 (1.38 to 2.01)	1.56 (1.18 to 2.05)
Amitriptyline ever	1.49 (1.15 to 1.94)	1.07 (0.70 to 1.66)
Dothiepin ever	1.73 (1.33 to 2.26)	1.67 (1.17 to 2.36)
Lofepramine ever	1.66 (1.13 to 2.44)	1.54 (0.81 to 2.93)

*Adjusted for diabetes, hypertension, body mass index, and smoking status, as well as the ever use of other types of antidepressants for each category.

Table 2. Additional results focusing on dothiepin

	No. of cases (n = 933)	No. of controls (n = 5516)	Adjusted odds ratio*	Test for trend, p value
Highest dose of dothiepin (mg)				
0	854	5228	1.00	
1 to 49	5	36	1.40	0.003
50 to 99	51	186	1.72	
⩾100	23	66	1.77	
No. of prescriptions of dothiepin				
0	854	5228	1.00	
1	19	72	1.52	0.002
2 or 3	18	69	1.39	
⩾4	28	81	1.96	

*Adjusted for hypertension, diabetes, body mass index, smoking status, and ever use of SSRI, amitriptyline, lofepramine and other antidepressants.

Question BI

(a)   What type of study is this?

[I mark]

(b)   Consider the results in the first table for 'SSRI ever' category.

(i)   Your SHO interpreted the unadjusted odds ratio of I.55 as "patients who took SSRI were expected to be I.55 times more likely to have a diagnosis of ischaemic heart disease". Is this accurate?

[I mark]

(ii)   Explain your answer.

[2 marks]

(iii)   The adjusted odds ratio for the 'SSRI ever' category is I.29 (0.89–I.87). What conclusions can you draw from the figure I.29?

[I mark]

(iv)   Is the result in question BIb(iii) above statistically significant? Explain your answer.

[I mark]

(v)   Why should the adjusted odds ratio be different from the unadjusted odds ratio?

[2 marks]

(vi)   What conclusion can you draw from this difference?

[2 marks]

Question B2

(a)   *Briefly* summarise the results of

(i)   unadjusted odds in Table I, ignoring the results for 'SSRI ever' category

[3 marks]

(ii)   adjusted odds in Table I, ignoring the results for the 'SSRI ever' category

[3 marks]

(b)   Name 2 variables other than those mentioned in the footnote of Table I which might be important to adjust for.

[2 marks each, up to a maximum of 4 marks]

Question B3

(a)   Briefly state the *two* main conclusions from the 'test for trend' results in Table 2.

[2 marks each, up to a maximum of 4 marks]

(b)
(i)   What is the main purpose of the analysis in Table 2?

[1 mark]

(ii)   How would you interpret the conclusions given in your answer to question B3a bearing in mind the purpose given in your answer to question B3b?

[1 mark]

(c)   Assuming that the study was properly carried out and analysed, what other evidence may be helpful to support the hypothesis that dothiepin causes ischaemic heart disease? (Give 2 points)

[1 mark each, up to maximum of 2 marks]

(d)   Give 2 alternative explanations for the significant association noted in part B2(a) of your answer other than that the relevant drug causes ischaemic heart disease.

[1 mark each, up to maximum of 2 marks]

Model answers by Mona Freeman

Question AI

(a)

(i) Advantage – Participants were more likely to comply with the follow-up study if only one assessment was required.

Disadvantage – No information can be gained as to the trends in the outcome variables over time since the intervention.

(ii) Advantage – This allows for sufficient time to look at the long-term effects of the intervention.

Disadvantage – A long interval between assessments increases the likelihood of participants being lost to follow-up.

(b)

Disadvantage – the assessors in the follow-up assessments were not blind to treatment group status, increasing the possibility of introducing a systematic experimenter bias.

Question A2

(a)

1. The participants were randomly allocated to the intervention or control groups.

2. The CBT arm was controlled for in terms of time and professional contact.

(b)

1. Was there adequate informed consent, given the severity of the participants' symptoms at the outset of the study?

2. The patients are likely to have not been blind to their treatment group status, increasing the chance of bias.

3. The criterion of 'acute psychosis' may produce a heterogeneous group including patients with different diagnoses, such as schizophrenia and drug-induced psychosis, which may have differing courses of responses to the intervention.

4. The CBT arm of the study included many different stages including family work; can one determine whether it was this, the group CBT or the individual CBT that actually had the effect?

5. There was no intention-to-treat analysis; the patients that dropped out should have been included in the analysis.

6. The study is small, it is not clear if a power calculation was done prior to the commencement of the study. As a result, there is an increased chance of a Type II error.

7. Many statistical tests were performed on the data, the data being subcategorised further for this, increasing the chances of a Type 1 error.

8. I would criticise the lack of confidence interval data presented – the s.d. gives no measure of precision, so you can't say what the range of population values might be.

Question A3

(a)

There were no significant differences between the CBT group and the recreation/informal support group at follow-up with regards to number of relapses, number of admissions, time in acute care or time to first relapse.

(b)

The data on relapses and readmissions are likely to be skewed (i.e. not normally distributed) because the given standard deviations are greater than the means. It is not possible to have negative values for these data.

(c)

There is a trend, although not significant, towards a longer time to first relapse in the CBT group compared with the control group, approximately $2\frac{1}{2}$ years compared with 1 year respectively. The use of the median as a descriptor implies that the data are skewed, not normally distributed. Clinically, this information means that long-term follow up is required over several years even if patients are symptom free, particularly in those who have had a CBT course.

Question A4

(a)
There were no significant differences in the outcome variables between the CBT group and the control group, although there was a consistent trend towards greater difficulties in the control group.

(b)
The subgroup results show, on the whole, significant ($p < 0.05$) differences between the CBT and the control group, with the control group having significantly increased rates of positive symptoms and delusions and significantly less perceived control over their illness.

(c)
Increasing the number of statistical tests performed on one set of data increases the chance of finding an aberrant significant result (a type I error).

(d)
In order to provide a conservative estimate of the effect of the intervention on delusions in the participants, so it was not overestimated.

(e)
They would have given the highest possible score for delusions to those from the CBT group and the lowest possible score for delusions to those from the control group.

Question A5

(a)
1. Have the rating scales been validated in a similar population to that being used in the study?

2. At what score does a particular variable become clinically significant?

(b)
Not necessarily. The level of difference needed to show statistical significance is arbitrarily set and based on probability. Some results which are not statistically significant (e.g. in this study – the median time to relapse) may be very clinically significant, to both patients and staff. Also, some statistically significant results may not be clinically important (e.g. the statistical difference in some outcomes from Table 2 may be irrelevant if the CBT patients still had levels of illness which interfered with their daily functioning).

(c)
Response – the absence of psychotic phenomena (delusions and hallucinations) on follow-up.

Response – not being readmitted to hospital in follow-up period.

Advantage – this would give you a dichotomous outcome, allowing you to calculate relative risks and numbers needed to treat (NNT).

Disadvantage – you need to reduce the data into a dichotomous outcome – you therefore need to define a clinically significant 'cut-off' for the outcome measures, which may be difficult especially with subjective, qualitative data such as the stigma/attitude to illness data, or other self-report measures.

Question A6

(a)
$40/8 = 5$ patients per week.

(b)
$5 \times 3 = 15$ rolling total. $5/15 = 1/3$ of the patients could be taken on for CBT.

(c)
1. You could employ more psychologists.

2. You could train other ward staff to be able to give the treatment such as senior nurses or nurse practitioners.

3. You could modify the treatment to include less individual and more group work – thus using the psychologist's time more efficiently.

Question A7

(a)

1. The study is not representative of our patients – different geographical area or demographics.

2. Our patients are frequent relapsers and as such are less likely to respond to this intervention.

3. This is expensive treatment and we have no extra money or resources to implement it.

4. This is a small study – we need more evidence, for example from similar studies in other populations that are sufficiently powered, to be sure that this is a true effect of CBT.

5. We do not know whether there are any adverse consequences of this treatment and would need to have more information about this before implementing it widely.

(b)

1. Patient satisfaction questionnaires.

2. Family satisfaction questionnaires.

3. DNA rates (patients not attending the CBT sessions or outpatient appointments).

4. Rates of readmission.

5. Length of hospital stay.

Question BI

(a)
Case–control study.

(b)
(i) No.

(ii) This is inaccurate because of the presence of numerous confounders, hence the calculation of the 'adjusted odds ratio' which takes account of these factors.

(iii) Patients in the sample who have had an SSRI, having adjusted for other variables, are on average 1.29 times more likely to also have a diagnosis of ischaemic heart disease than not, when compared with those who have not had an SSRI. However, in the population, 95% of patients who have had an SSRI are between 0.89 and 1.87 times more likely to have this diagnosis.

(iv) No. Not statistically significant because the confidence interval crosses 1 (unity, the value where there is no difference between the odds in either group).

(v) It is different because of the additional effect of confounding factors (diabetes, BMI, smoking, etc.), which will also – independent of the use of SSRIs – increase the likelihood of a diagnosis of ischaemic heart disease.

(vi) When considered alone, the use of SSRIs does not significantly increase the likelihood of also having a diagnosis of ischaemic heart disease, but the use of SSRIs is associated with an increased frequency of other known risk factors for the disease.

Question B2

(a)
(i) Without adjusting for confounders, overall, patients exposed to tricyclic antidepressants are significantly more likely to also have a diagnosis of IHD than not, when compared with patients not exposed to TCAs. Of the TCAs studied, dothiepin exposure is most likely to be significantly associated with IHD (1.73 times more likely), followed by lofepramine (1.66 times more likely) and then amitriptyline (1.49 times more likely).

(ii) When one takes account of the confounding factors mentioned, overall, patients exposed to TCAs remain significantly more likely to have a diagnosis of IHD, albeit at a lower level than when not separating out the other risk factors – 1.56 times compared with 1.67 times. However, dothiepin is now the sole specific TCA studied which remains significantly associated with a diagnosis of IHD.

(b)
Age. Family history of IHD.

Question B3

(a)
The chance of having a diagnosis of IHD increases significantly as the dose of dothiepin one is exposed to increases and as the total lifetime exposure to dothiepin (measured by the number of prescriptions) increases.

(b)
(i) To assess whether dothiepin may be a causative factor for the development of IHD rather than just an associated factor.

(ii) Dothiepin can cause IHD.

(c)
1. A logical biological/pharmacological hypothesis or link between dothiepin and IHD.

2. Supportive evidence from other studies (for example animal studies) or those on a different population.

(d)
1. Depression causes ischaemic heart disease.

2. Alternatively, the association is explained by another uncontrolled-for confounder such as age – which can be associated with both IHD and dothiepin exposure.

MRCPsych Part II Examination
Critical Review Paper
Spring 2004

Please read the instructions carefully before going further.

Instructions

1. This examination lasts for 90 minutes.
2. The paper has TWO questions, Question A and Question B, *each of which should be answered using separate answer booklets as indicated.*
3. You must *attempt* ALL parts of BOTH questions.
4. A total of 100 marks has been allocated to the whole paper. Each part of each question is worth 10 marks. Therefore, Question A is worth 70 marks, and Question B is worth 30 marks.
5. In answering Question A, candidates may wish to glance briefly at the questions they are asked to answer (on pages 142–146 of the paper), before reading the details of the research (described on pages 140–142).
6. Where you give more than the requested number of answers, you will only be marked on that number, e.g. If you are asked for 5 examples and give 6, you will only be marked on the first 5.
7. Candidates are advised to bring a calculator to the examination hall for this paper. Candidates are only permitted to take a noiseless, cordless, pocket-sized non-programmable calculator WITHOUT printout or graphic/word display facilities.
8. Please do not remove this Examination paper from the Examination Room.

Question A

Low dose tricyclics

As an SHO in psychiatry, you see a 40-year-old woman referred by the general practitioner with a classic history of moderately severe acute depression for the past 3 months. Her general practitioner has diagnosed the condition correctly and prescribed amitriptyline 75 mg daily. You present the history to your consultant and she asks you to write to the general practitioner, to say that perhaps this patient has been undertreated and that treatment of adult depression with such a low dose of tricyclic antidepressant can be hard to justify.

As you are about to send your letter to the general practitioner, you suddenly come across the following systematic review:

Furukawa, T.A., McGuire, H., Barbui, C. Meta-analysis of effects and side effects of low dosage tricyclic antidepressants in depression: systematic review. *BMJ* 2002; **325**: 991–995.

The paper

The objectives of this systematic review are to compare the effects and side-effects of low dosage tricyclic antidepressants with placebo and with standard dosage tricyclics in acute phase of depression.

Methods

The systematic review includes randomised trials, lasting at least 4 weeks, comparing low dosage tricyclics with placebo, or with standard dosages of the same tricyclic in adults with acute depression. Low dosage was defined as 100 mg/day or less of imipramine, amitriptyline, clomipramine, desipramine, doxepin, dothiepin, trimipramine, or lofepramine. The primary outcome was the effect of treatment on depression, according to the original authors' definition, but usually defined as 50% or greater reduction in severity of depression. The severity of symptoms was measured by either observer rating or self-report.

The authors electronically searched the Cochrane Collaboration depression, anxiety, and neurosis controlled trials register up to November 2000 for any trials in which tricyclics were given. Potential papers were examined manually by two reviewers and then checked according to the strict eligibility criteria by two reviewers independently. To identify further trials, references of these selected studies and of other review papers were also checked, representative studies were subjected to SciSearch, and authors and experts were contacted.

The methodological quality of the selected studies was assessed. Data were extracted by two reviewers independently. Disagreements between them were resolved by consensus.

Heterogeneity between studies was assessed both statistically and by visual inspection of the results.

Results

Of 2,418 citations originally identified, 141 were potentially relevant. The authors agreed on 35 studies (2,013 participants) that compared low dosage tricyclics with placebo and 6 studies (551 participants) that compared low dosage tricyclics with standard dosage tricyclics. The kappas (which measure inter-rater reliability) for the assessment for eligibility and validity were between 0.58 and 0.86.

Sixteen studies used amitriptyline as active drugs and 13 used imipramine. Ten studies were conducted in primary care and 12 studies in psychiatric settings. Six studies dealt with depression seen in patients with co-morbid physical conditions (e.g. migraine, rheumatoid arthritis). There were enough details on the randomisation procedure in four of the studies.

Low dosage tricyclics versus placebo

The relative risk of a response for low dosage tricyclics compared to placebo at 4 weeks and 6–8 weeks were 1.65 (95% CI 1.36–2.00) and 1.47 (95% CI 1.12–1.94) respectively. The apparent advantage of low dosage tricyclics was not maintained when intention to treat analysis based on the worst case scenario was carried out. When analyses were carried out based on continuous measures, people taking low dosage tricyclics had scores for severity of depression that were 0.59 (95% CI 0.30–0.87) and 0.59 (95% CI 0.20–0.99) standard deviations lower than those taking placebo at 4 weeks and 6–8 weeks respectively.

The relative risk of dropouts, whatever their causes, of the lower dosage tricyclics compared to placebo groups was 1.08 (95% CI 0.93–1.26). Overall, 24% of enrolled participants dropped out by the end of the trial. People taking low dosage tricyclics were 111% (95% CI 35%–228%) more likely than those taking placebo to drop out *due to side effects*.

The funnel plot showed some asymmetry in that the five smallest studies reported large relative risks in favour of low dosage tricyclics. These studies mainly dated from the 1960s and 1970s and involved patients recruited outside a clinical setting. When they were omitted, the funnel plot was symmetrical and the relative risks decreased only slightly to 1.58 (95% CI 1.31 to 1.90) at 4 weeks and 1.28 (95% CI 1.05 to 1.55) at 6–8 weeks.

Low dosage tricyclics vs standard dosage tricyclics

The relative risk for responses at 4 weeks and 6–8 weeks are shown in figure 1 below. Note that in the second and third columns, N stands for the number of subjects and n stands for the number of responders in the relevant arm of each study. Low dosage tricyclics were 55% (95% CI 24%–73%) less likely than standard dose tricyclics to cause dropouts due to side effects.

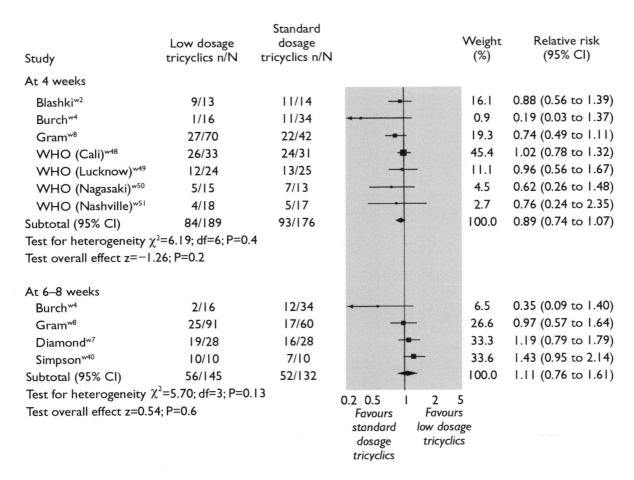

Study	Low dosage tricyclics n/N	Standard dosage tricyclics n/N		Weight (%)	Relative risk (95% CI)
At 4 weeks					
Blashki[w2]	9/13	11/14		16.1	0.88 (0.56 to 1.39)
Burch[w4]	1/16	11/34		0.9	0.19 (0.03 to 1.37)
Gram[w8]	27/70	22/42		19.3	0.74 (0.49 to 1.11)
WHO (Cali)[w48]	26/33	24/31		45.4	1.02 (0.78 to 1.32)
WHO (Lucknow)[w49]	12/24	13/25		11.1	0.96 (0.56 to 1.67)
WHO (Nagasaki)[w50]	5/15	7/13		4.5	0.62 (0.26 to 1.48)
WHO (Nashville)[w51]	4/18	5/17		2.7	0.76 (0.24 to 2.35)
Subtotal (95% CI)	84/189	93/176		100.0	0.89 (0.74 to 1.07)
Test for heterogeneity χ^2=6.19; df=6; P=0.4					
Test overall effect z=−1.26; P=0.2					
At 6–8 weeks					
Burch[w4]	2/16	12/34		6.5	0.35 (0.09 to 1.40)
Gram[w8]	25/91	17/60		26.6	0.97 (0.57 to 1.64)
Diamond[w7]	19/28	16/28		33.3	1.19 (0.79 to 1.79)
Simpson[w40]	10/10	7/10		33.6	1.43 (0.95 to 2.14)
Subtotal (95% CI)	56/145	52/132		100.0	1.11 (0.76 to 1.61)
Test for heterogeneity χ^2=5.70; df=3; P=0.13					
Test overall effect z=0.54; P=0.6					

Figure 1.

Question A1

The authors tried to answer their research questions by performing a systematic review rather than a new large randomised controlled trial. Give

(a)   four advantages

(b)   six disadvantages

of a systematic review compared to a new large randomised controlled trial to address the authors' questions.

[1 mark for each advantage and disadvantage, up to a maximum of 10 marks]

Question A2

(a)   *Briefly* explain how publication bias might occur.

[1 mark]

(b)   In a funnel plot, what is on the x-axis (i.e. horizontal axis)?

[1 mark]

What is on the y-axis (i.e. vertical axis)?

[1 mark]

(c)   What shape of a funnel plot might suggest

(i)   an absence of publication bias

(ii)   the presence of publication bias?

In each case, briefly explain how such shapes may arise.

[1 mark each up to a maximum of 2 marks]

(d)   Name one way in which the authors

(i)   minimised publication bias

(ii)   tested for publication bias

(iii)   minimised selection bias after the studies have been identified.

[1 mark for each part, up to a maximum of 3 marks]

(e)   Name two potential sources of bias in identifying published studies.

[1 mark each up to a maximum of 2 marks]

Question A3

(a)   The authors stated that the two reviewers examined papers and then independently checked according to the strict eligibility criteria. List 3 eligibility criteria which have been used in this meta-analysis.

[1 mark each, up to a maximum of 3 marks]

(b)   Having identified studies which satisfy the strict eligibility criteria, the reviewers then assess the methodological quality of these selected studies. Name 4 criteria which the reviewers were likely to have used to assess methodological quality.

[1 mark each, up to a maximum of 4 marks]

(c)   Look at the figure relating to data at 4 weeks. Examine the data on the two studies by WHO (Cali) and WHO (Nagasaki). More weight is placed on the former study (45.4%) than the latter (4.5%). How would you explain this observation?

[3 marks]

Question A4

(a)   The kappas for the assessment for eligibility and validity were between 0.58 and 0.86. *Briefly interpret these figures.*

[2 marks]

(b)   The relative risk of a response for low dosage tricyclics compared to placebo at 4 weeks was 1.65 (95% CI 1.36–2.00). What conclusion would you draw from this result?

[2 marks]

(c)   The authors stated that 'apparent advantage of low dosage tricyclics was not maintained when intention to treat analysis based on the worst case scenario was carried out'.

(i)   Briefly explain what is meant by 'intention to treat analysis based on the worst case scenario'.

[2 marks]

(ii)   Would the results be likely to show more advantage, no change, or even less advantage for low dosage tricyclics if the overall dropout rate were 40% rather than 24%?

[1 mark]

(d)
(i)   Interpret the result given for response to low dosage tricyclics compared to placebo at 4 weeks when analysis was carried out *based on continuous measures*. Briefly explain your answer.

[2 marks]

(ii)   Are these results consistent with your answers to part (b) above?

[1 mark]

Question A5

(a)   What conclusion can you draw from the result on the relative risk of dropouts, whatever their causes, of the lower dosage tricyclics compared to placebo groups?

[1 mark]

(b)   What is the relative risk (and 95% confidence interval) of dropouts *due to side effects* of the lower dosage tricyclics compared to placebo groups?

[3 marks]

(c)

(i)   'The funnel plot showed some asymmetry in that the five smallest studies reported large relative risks in favour of low dosage tricyclics'. What conclusion would you draw from this statement alone?

[2 marks]

(ii)   'These studies mainly dated from the 1960s and 1970s and involved patients recruited outside a clinical setting. When they were omitted, the funnel plot was symmetrical.'

A.   Give one conclusion the authors implicitly invite the readers to draw from this finding.

[2 marks]

B.   Briefly explain whether you agree with the implicit conclusion in your answer to A. above.

[2 marks]

Question A6

(a)   Briefly explain what is meant by

(i)   clinical heterogeneity

[1 mark]

(ii)   statistical heterogeneity.

[1 mark]

(b)   List 2 pieces of information given in the summary which might result in clinical heterogeneity.

[1 mark each, up to a maximum of 2 marks]

(c)   Examine figure 1. Using two separate methods, deduce whether there is statistical heterogeneity in the studies comparing low dosage tricyclics with standard dosage tricyclics at 4 weeks. Explain each method briefly.

[4 marks]

(d)
(i)   Generally, is it possible for there to be statistical heterogeneity without clinical heterogeneity?

(ii)   Generally, is it possible for there to be clinical heterogeneity without statistical heterogeneity?

[1 mark each, up to a maximum of 2 marks]

Question A7

(a)   Briefly list three conclusions on the effectiveness and the side effects comparing low dosage tricyclics with standard dosage tricyclics.

[2 marks each, total 6 marks]

(b)   Your consultant said that "treatment of adult depression with such a low dose of tricyclic antidepressants can be hard to justify". After having read this paper, is the opinion of your consultant that adult depression should not be treated with a low dose tricyclic antidepressant justified?

[1 mark]

Give three points for your answer.

[1 mark each up to a maximum of 3 marks]

Question B

The following figure is taken from a paper which studied the prevalence of and risk factors for clinical hypothyroidism in patients treated with lithium carbonate. (Johnston A. M. & Eagles, J. M. Lithium-associated clinical hypothyroidism. Prevalence and risk factors. *British Journal of Psychiatry*, 1999; **175**: 336–339).

   The authors examined the time to onset of clinical hypothyroidism after the onset of continuous lithium treatment in men and women. Of 430 women and 265 men on lithium and who were having thyroxine and TSH (thyroid stimulating hormone) estimations, 341 women (79%) and 207 men (78%) were followed up. The figure shows the relationship between survival to hypothyroidism and months on continuous lithium.

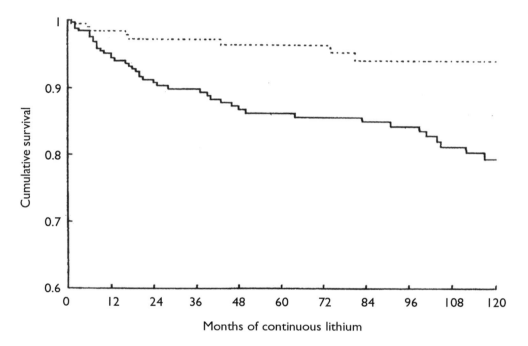

Figure 1. Ten-year survival for 'time to hypothyroidism' in women *v.* men: (······) men, $n=207$ at start; (——) women, $n=341$ at start.

Question BI

(a)   Interpret what the figure shows.

[4 marks]

(b)   What do the horizontal sections on the survival curves mean?

[2 marks]

(c)
(i)   What do the steps in the survival curves mean?

[2 marks]

(ii)   Explain your answer.

[2 marks]

Question B2

(a)   Estimate the time to median survival for each group.

[2 marks]

(b)   Studies of this type are known as survival analyses.

(i)   How may development of hypothyroidism not be detected? Give 2 examples.

[2 marks for each, up to a maximum of 4 marks]

(ii)   Estimate the relative risk of hypothyroidism of women compared to men at 10 years.

[2 marks]

(iii)   If a woman is free from hypothyroidism at 2 years, what is the chance of her remaining free from hypothyroidism for another 3 years (i.e. at 5 years)?

[2 marks]

Question B3

Give 5 points that you need to know in general to conclude that the use of lithium causes clinical hypothyroidism.

[2 marks for each, up to a maximum of 10 marks]

Model answers by Anne-Marie Feeley

Question A1

Four advantages of a systematic review:

1. A systematic review is much cheaper to conduct than a large RCT.

2. A systematic review, by summarising the results of many different studies, will possibly yield more accurate information on which are the most effective treatments than a single RCT.

3. The results of a systematic review may be mathematically collated into a meta-analysis, giving a precise summary effect-size. A meta-analysis based on a comprehensive systematic review is the gold standard of evidence-based medicine.

4. A systematic review can explore and interpret possible heterogeneity of findings in different studies.

Six disadvantages of a systematic review:

A systematic review may be prone to a variety of biases:

1. Language bias (choosing only English-language studies).

2. Selection bias (e.g. using just one database such as Medline will give you only approximately 40% of the available information. Several databases should be searched).

3. Publication bias (negative studies are much less likely to be published).

4. In a systematic review, it is not possible to set your own eligibility criteria or outcome measures.

5. The systematic review will be limited by the quality of the included studies.

6. Different studies may have different end-points, and so it may be very difficult to compare and collate them for the purposes of a review.

Question A2

(a)
Studies that yield positive results are much more likely to be accepted for publication. Small, negative studies are by contrast unlikely to be published.

(b)
In a funnel plot, the x-axis shows the size of the effect.

The y-axis shows the size of the study sample.

(c)
(i) If there is no publication bias, there will be an even spread of results (both positive and negative) around the true effect-size, giving a symmetrical funnel-shaped curve.

(ii) If publication bias has occurred, you would expect to see a 'hole' in the expected funnel shape where the small, negative trials (which are trials least likely to be published) should be. If publication bias has occurred, the curve will no longer be symmetrical.

(d)
(i) The authors minimised publication bias by checking the references of the studies they selected.

(ii) They tested for publication bias by using a funnel plot (which showed a publication bias toward positive studies).

(iii) The selected studies were each assessed independently by two reviewers to ensure that they met the strict eligibility criteria for inclusion in the systematic review.

(e)
Potential sources of bias in identifying published studies:

1. Selection bias (searching only one database).

2. Language bias.

Question A3

(a)
The eligibility criteria the authors used are:

1. Trials must be randomised.

2. They must be of at least 4 weeks' duration.

3. The trials selected compared either low-dosage tricyclics with placebo, or low-dosage tricyclics with standard-dose tricyclics.

(b)
1. The study sample chosen should be representative of the population of interest. (Theoretically, if you are conducting a study on patients with schizophrenia, then every single person with that illness, whether they are in treatment or not, should have an equal chance of being included in the study.)

2. The subjects should be allocated randomly to each arm of the study.

3. Gold standard measures should be used both to ascertain diagnoses and measure response.

4. The subjects should be blinded as to which treatment they are receiving. (This is difficult to do in studies on psychotherapy, and also if the active drug in a placebo-controlled trial has very marked or obvious side-effects.)

(c)
Weighting of studies is based on three main factors: the relative size, quality and external validity of each study.

The WHO (Cali) trial has a large sample size and a narrow confidence interval, indicating that its results are likely to be accurate. In contrast, the WHO (Nagasaki) study has a very small sample size and a very wide confidence interval, indicating that its results are not likely to be very accurate.

In addition to sample size, the authors would also take into account the relative quality of each study: it is possible the WHO (Cali) study was of higher quality than the WHO (Nagasaki) study. Owing to its large size, it may also be more representative, therefore scoring higher for external validity.

Question A4

(a)
A kappa score is a measure of inter-rater reliability. It measures the degree of agreement between two raters, taking into account the agreement that would occur by chance. A kappa score of 0.80 or above indicates good agreement.

Agreement varied from 0.58 to 0.86, which means that for some studies there was very good agreement between raters as to eligibility and validity (kappa of 0.86), and for others the agreement was poor (kappa of 0.58).

(b)
Subjects on low-dosage tricyclics were 1.65 times more likely to respond at 4 weeks than those on placebo. This result is statistically significant (P=0.05), because the confidence interval does not cross 1.

(c)
(i) An 'intention to treat analysis based on worst case scenario' means that the researchers presumed that of all those subjects who dropped out of the study before it was completed, those in the active-treatment group did badly and all those in the control (placebo) group did well. They then included these results in their final analysis.

(ii) More advantage.

(d)
(i) People taking low-dosage tricyclics did better at 4 weeks than those on placebo based on continuous measures, but not significantly so. This means that those on tricyclics had a bigger drop in their depression scores than those on placebo, but this was not significant at the P=0.05 level.

(ii) The results are measuring different things. In (b), we are talking about response, defined as a 50% reduction in the severity of depression, whereas in (d) we are talking about a drop in depression scores, which is a slightly different thing. Tricyclics were better than placebo when measuring response and when looking at drops in depression scores; the only difference is that the first measure reached statistical significance at the P=0.05 level, and the second did not.

Question A5

(a)

There is no significant difference in the relative risk of drop-outs in the tricyclic vs. the placebo group, because the 95% CI crosses 1.

(b)

The relative risk of dropping out in the tricyclic group due to side effects is 1.11 compared with placebo.

The 95% CI is 0.35–2.28.

(c)

(i)   This means that there is publication bias, with a lack of small negative studies.

(ii)

A. They suggest that these small studies were possibly of poor quality, out-dated and with unrepresentative subjects, and so were likely to have yielded inaccurate results.

B. I think the authors are correct in making these assumptions, given that these studies yielded aberrant results, and that their removal from the review did not alter the overall results significantly.

Question A6

(a)

(i)   Clinical heterogeneity occurs when the subjects chosen for two studies differ from one another significantly, making the results of these studies difficult to collate.

(ii) Statistical heterogeneity occurs when the results of different studies differ from one another significantly more than would be expected by chance.

(b)

1.   Some studies were based in primary care, while others took place in psychiatric settings. (It is likely that those in primary care had less severe depression, making the two groups clinically heterogeneous.)

2.   Some studies looked at depression occurring in patients with physical illnesses; again, these patients may be significantly different from patients with depression but without comorbid illnesses.

(c)

Visual inspection of the studies as shown in Figure 1 is one way of checking for heterogeneity. In general, the studies give fairly similar results, with only the small study by Burch yielding markedly different results from the average. This suggests that there is no significant heterogeneity.

Heterogeneity can also be measured using statistical means, as shown in Figure 1. In this case, the statistical tests for heterogeneity yielded a P-value of 0.4, which is not significant.

A funnel plot could be drawn from these studies and adapted to test for heterogeneity by using different symbols for different types of studies (e.g. those studies which used amitriptyline could be plotted using a different symbol from those using imipramine). If studies with the same symbols aggregate together, it is likely to be due to heterogeneity.

(d)

(i)   Yes. Two studies could be measuring the same thing in similar populations, but by using different methodologies could come up with different results.

(ii) Yes. Two studies could be measuring the same thing in very different populations, but could still come up with very similar results.

Question A7

(a)

1.   Those on low-dosage tricyclics were significantly less likely to drop out because of side-effects than those on standard doses at the 95% confidence level.

2.   At 4 weeks, approx. 53% of people on standard-dose tricyclics had responded, compared with approx. 44% of those on low-dose tricyclics, based on the pooled results of all the studies. However, this difference was not statistically significant, as the confidence interval for the pooled effect-size includes 1.

3.   At 6–8 weeks, there were no significant differences in the two treatments when the results were pooled, with a wide confidence interval of 0.76–1.61.

(b)

No.

1. Low-dose tricyclics appear to be more acceptable in terms of side-effect profile.

2. There are no significant differences in response rates based on these studies at 4 weeks.

3. There are no significant differences in response rates at 6–8 weeks.

Question B1

(a)
The figure shows, from a group of 341 women (represented by the dark line) and 207 men (represented by the dotted line), how many patients on continuous lithium treatment developed hypothyroidism over a period of 10 years after commencing the drug. (Or, to put it another way, how many patients 'survived', i.e. did not develop hypothyroidism despite being on lithium for 10 years.)

(b)
The horizontal sections represent periods of time in which no one developed hypothyroidism. (This could also be expressed as periods of time in which the prevalence of hypothyroidism in the study group remained constant.)

(c)
(i) & (ii) Each step in the survival curve shows a drop in the cumulative survival of the study sample, and represents the proportion of the study sample that developed hypothyroidism at that point in time.

Question B2

Women: 25 years
Men: 100 years
Median survival rate is the length of time that 50% of the population survived without the outcome of interest occurring (in this case, hypothyroidism).

(b)
(i)
1. Some patients may develop hypothyroidism after 10 years, and so would not be detected in this study.

2. Only 79% of women and 78% of men were followed up; we do not know whether or not those who were not followed up developed hypothyroidism.

(ii) Relative risk is the risk of the outcome in women divided by the risk of the outcome in men at 10 years.
   The risk in women is the number of women who become hypothyroid out of the total number of women in the study: this is 20%, according to the graph. The risk for men is 5%.
   The relative risk is 4: women are four times more likely to develop hypothyroidism than men over 10 years of lithium therapy.

(iii) At 2 years (24 months), this woman is one of the 90% of women who are free of hypothyroidism. By 5 years (60 months), another 5% will have developed hypothyroidism. This woman has just a 5% chance of developing the illness in the next 3 years, so has a 95% chance of staying well at 5 years.

Question B3

1. People taking lithium should be at significantly increased risk compared with the general population of becoming hypothyroid. We need to know the prevalence of hypothyroidism in the general population before we can say that the risk is increased on lithium.

2. There should be a dose–response relationship between the two, i.e. the longer you have been on lithium, and the higher the dose, the more likely you are to become hypothyroid in the future.

3. There should be a temporal relationship between taking lithium and becoming hypothyroid, i.e. you must be sure that the hypothyroidism did not precede the commencement of lithium.

4. The link should be consistent with existing knowledge; e.g. replication of the association in different studies.

5. Reversibility: stopping lithium should reverse the hypothyroidism.

Reference list of papers used in the examinations

Anderson, C., Connelly, J., Johnstone, E. C., *et al* (1991) Disabilities and circumstances of schizophrenic patients – a follow-up study. V. Cause of death. *British Journal of Psychiatry,* **159** (suppl. 13), 30–33.

Angold, A., Costello, E. J., Farmer, E. M., *et al* (1999) Impaired but undiagnosed. *Journal of the American Academy of Child and Adolescent Psychiatry,* **38**, 129–137.

Boardman, A. P., Grimbaldeston, A. H., Handley, C., *et al* (1999) The North Staffordshire suicide study: a case–control study of suicide in one health district. *Psychological Medicine,* **29**, 27–33.

Bowden, C. L., Brugger, A. M., Swann, A. C., *et al* (1994) Efficacy of divalproex *vs* lithium and placebo in the treatment of mania. *JAMA,* **271**, 918–924.

Bower, P., Byford, S., Sibbald, B., *et al* (2000) Randomised controlled trial of non-directive counselling, cognitive–behaviour therapy, and usual general practitioner care for patients with depression. II: cost effectiveness. *BMJ,* **321**, 1389–1392.

Drury, V., Birchwood, M. & Cochrane, R. (2000) Cognitive therapy and recovery from acute psychosis: a controlled trial. *British Journal of Psychiatry,* **177**, 8–14.

Fava, G. A., Rafanelli, C., Grandi, S., *et al* (1998) Prevention of recurrent depression with cognitive behavioral therapy: preliminary findings. *Archives of General Psychiatry,* **55**, 816–820.

Fleming, M. F., Barry, K. L., Manwell, L. B., *et al* (1997) Brief physician advice for problem alcohol drinkers. A randomised controlled trial in community-based primary care practices. *Journal of the American Medical Association,* **277**, 1039–1045.

Furukawa, T. A., McGuire, H. & Barbui, C. (2002) Meta-analysis of effects and side effects of low dosage tricyclic antidepressants in depression: systematic review. *BMJ,* **325**, 991–995.

Garland, M., Hickey, D., Corvin, A., *et al* (2000) Total serum cholesterol in relation to psychological correlates in parasuicide. *British Journal of Psychiatry,* **177**, 77–83.

Hippisley-Cox, J., Pringle, M., Hammersley, V., *et al* (2001) Antidepressants as risk factor for ischaemic heart disease: case–control study in primary care. *BMJ,* **323**, 666–669.

Johnstone, A. M. & Eagles, J. M. (1999) Lithium-associated clinical hypothyroidism. *British Journal of Psychiatry,* **175**, 336–339.

Kessler, D., Lloyd, K., Lewis, G., *et al* (1999) Cross sectional study of symptom attribution and recognition of depression and anxiety in primary care. *British Medical Journal,* **318**, 436–439.

Lindberg, G., Bingefors, K., Ranstam, J., *et al* (1998) Use of calcium channel blockers and risk of suicide: ecological findings confirmed in population based cohort study. *BMJ,* **316**, 741–745.

Mason, P., Harrison, G., Glazebrook, C., *et al* (1995) Characteristics of outcome in schizophrenia at 13 years. *British Journal of Psychiatry,* **167**, 596–603.

Mayou, R. A., Ehlers, A. & Hobbs, M. (2000) Psychological debriefing for road traffic accident victims. Three-year follow-up of a randomised controlled trial. *British Journal of Psychiatry,* **176**, 589–593.

Nandy, S., Chalmers-Watson, C., Gantley, M., *et al* (2001) Referral for minor mental illness: a qualitative study. *British Journal of General Practice,* **51**, 461–465.

Pulska, T., Pahkala, K., Laippala, P., *et al* (1999) Follow up study of longstanding depression as predictor of mortality in elderly people living in the community. *BMJ*, **318**, 432–433.

Sadowski, H., Ugarte, B., Kolvin, I., *et al* (1999) Early life family disadvantages and major depression in adulthood. *British Journal of Psychiatry*, **174**, 112–120.

Viguera, A. C., Nonacs, R., Cohen, L. S., *et al* (2000) Risk of recurrence of bipolar disorder in pregnant and nonpregnant women after discontinuing lithium maintenance. *American Journal of Psychiatry*, **157**, 179–184.

Ward, E., King, M., Lloyd, M., *et al* (2000) Randomised controlled trial of non-directive counselling, cognitive–behaviour therapy, and usual general practitioner care for patients with depression. I: clinical effectiveness. *BMJ*, **321**, 1383–1388.

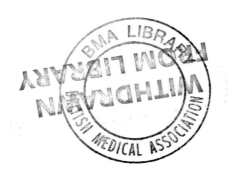